W0227700

Endoscopic Sinus Surgery

A Practical Approach

Springer-Verlag London Ltd.

S.K. Kaluskar
With a Contribution by Professor T. Ohinishi

Endoscopic Sinus Surgery

A Practical Approach

Foreword by Professor W. Draf

With 232 illustrations, 196 in colour

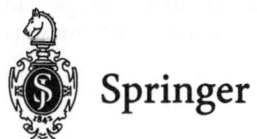 Springer

S.K. Kaluskar, MS, FRCS, DLO (Eng)
Consultant Otorhinolaryngologist, Tyrone County Hospital, Omagh,
Northern Ireland, UK

Contribution by
Toshio Ohinishi, MD
Department of Otolaryngology, St Luke's International Hospital,
Tokyo, Japan

British Library Cataloguing in Publication Data
Kaluskar, S.K.
Endoscopic sinus surgery: a practical approach
1. Paranasal sinuses – Endoscopic surgery
I. Title
617.5'23

ISBN 978-1-4471-1235-8   ISBN 978-1-4471-0919-8 (eBook)
DOI 10.1007/978-1-4471-0919-8

Library of Congress Cataloging-in-Publication Data
Kaluskar, S.K.
Endoscopic sinus surgery: a practical approach/S.K. Kaluskar.
p.   cm.
Includes bibliographical references and index.

1. Paranasal sinuses – Endoscopic surgery. I. Title.
[DNLM: 1. Paranasal Sinus Diseases – surgery. 2. Surgery,
Endoscopic – methods. 3. Paranasal Sinuses – anatomy & histology.
WV 340 K14e 1996]
RF421.K35 1996
617.5'23 – dc20
DNLM/DLC
for Library of Congress   96-17383

Apart from any fair dealing for the purposes of research or private study, or criticism or review, as permitted under the Copyright, Designs and Patents Act 1988, this publication may only reproduced, stored or transmitted, in any form or by any means, with the prior permission in writing of the publishers, or in the case of reprographic reproduction in accordance with the terms of licences issued by the Copyright Licensing Agency. Enquiries concerning reproduction outside those terms should be sent to the publishers.

© Springer-Verlag London 1997
Originally published by Springer-Verlag London Limited in 1997
Softcover reprint of the hardcover 1st edition 1997

The use of registered names, trademarks, etc. in this publication does not imply, even in the absence of a specific statement, that such names are exempt from the relevant laws and regulations and therefore free for general use.

Product liability: The publisher can give no guarantee for information about drug dosage and application thereof contained in this book. In every individual case the respective user must check its accuracy by consulting other pharmaceutical literature.

Typeset by EXPO Holdings, Malaysia

28/3830-543210 Printed on acid-free paper

Dedicated to
my wife, Hema, and children Komal, Anup and Soniya
who made it all worthwhile

Foreword

Ear, nose and throat surgeons all over the world remember well the evolution of ear surgery in the early fifties, when the concept of tympanoplasty was developed, providing cure for disease and its possible complications, and functional restoration of sound transmission of the middle ear. In a similar way, diagnosis and surgery of inflammatory diseases of paranasal sinuses had undergone basic changes within the last 20 years.

Endoscopy of the nose and paranasal sinuses was the first step, more extended surgery became safer and the first attempts at endoscopic surgery were made. Techniques for endo-nasal exploration of the paranasal sinuses had been described at the turn of the twentieth century but were soon abandoned because of frequent, severe complications. However, new visual aids such as the microscope and endoscope, a remarkable improvement in local and general anaesthesia, and an increasing reluctance of patients to accept the surgical sequelae of "radical" sinus procedures with almost total removal of mucosal lining all provided the impetus for a renaissance in endo-nasal practice.

The concept of functional endoscopic sinus surgery was first developed in Austria and Germany as a result of detailed studies of the physiology and pathology of the muco-ciliary transport mechanism. It facilitated the smallest possible intervention and the removal of severely diseased parts of mucosa, preservation of mucosa showing reversible pathology, and establishment of optimal drainage of all sinuses into the nose via an endo-nasal route. Functional endoscopic sinus surgery had gained overwhelming acceptance throughout the world by the mid 1980s.

Mr Kaluskar realised the importance of functional endoscopic sinus surgery at an early stage and the present monograph is the result of his diligent research and hard work in the field of this modern rhinosurgical technique, and his experience with a total of 532 operated cases and 1022 procedures. After intensive studies of the related anatomical structures, he started using mainly the technique of the Graz Messerklinger school, and restricting the more extended surgery of Wigand to severe cases and revisions. From the beginning he collected all the relevant data from his cases, which were processed by computer and analysed. He also developed modifications as, for example, combined approach middle meatal antrostomy (CAMMA).

This book is written for the beginner, describing step by step the route one has to follow until surgery may be started, the surgical technique itself, including some modifications and many "tricks". Chapter 14 (Tips for Beginners) makes clear why the old chestnut "practice makes perfect" is not good advice to the initiate in functional endoscopic sinus surgery. The discussion "Headaches and Facial Pains" is of utmost interest.

The final chapter, "Broadening the Horizons", gives a stimulating outlook for endo-nasal endoscopic sinus surgery. This publication is richly illustrated. The layout allows important points to be brought to the reader's particular attention. Appendix A shows the necessary equipment, and Appendix B supplies the necessary information for prospective documentation. With its meticulous review of results and complications, pitfalls and their prevention, this work will give significant support to the less experienced surgeon and cautions him or her of the possible dangers. For the advanced sinus surgeon seeking another experts opinion there is a rich mine of "tricks" and advice. We hope, this monograph will also stimulate head and neck and ear, nose and throat surgeons to expand their diagnostic as well as therapeutic abilities, and to improve the results of surgical management of patients with inflammatory paranasal sinus diseases.

Professor W. Draf
Director, University ENT Clinic, Fulda, Germany

Preface

The management of chronic inflammatory paranasal sinus disease has been transformed by an increasingly clear understanding of the pathophysiology of muco-ciliary clearance, the application of nasal endoscopy, both diagnostic and therapeutic and by recent developments in imaging techniques. Endoscopic sinus surgery (ESS) is a minimally invasive technique for the treatment of chronic sinus disease with significantly superior results.

This is a practical textbook on endoscopic sinus surgery with an emphasis on the basics of surgical anatomy, pathophysiology and, most importantly, endoscopic diagnosis; the surgeon must first diagnose the disease before he or she can treat, let alone operate! The book is intended not only for the practising ear, nose and throat and head and neck surgeons but also for trainees who will be able to enhance their understanding of the clinical presentation of chronic paranasal sinus disease and its management.

Information on the subject, surprisingly, is scarce, and falls mainly into two categories. Most standard ENT textbooks gloss over ESS, mentioning some historical aspects and basic techniques. The few books dealing specifically with the subject (they can almost be counted on the fingers of one hand!) assume a basic grasp of the topic on the part of the reader, and could pose difficulties for those who have limited or only recent access to endoscopy. There is, in my opinion, a need for a primer that provides a basic, visual overview of the why, the when and the how (*including the how not!*) of ESS.

This book takes the reader on a tour of the nose and sinuses in both health and disease, stopping to dwell on the intricacies of the ostio-meatal complex. Pre-operative evaluation using nasal endoscopy and computed tomography is discussed and illustrated. The surgical protocol is described step by step, as is post-operative care. Complications, and how to prevent and deal with them, are of particular importance in ESS. Since the surgeon is often operating millimetres away from the orbit and skull base, an intimate knowledge of anatomy gained in the dissection hall is of paramount value. Accordingly, numerous cadaveric and surgical illustrations are included.

I would like to emphasise my belief that nasal endoscopy is a very useful diagnostic procedure in its own right, and I would recommend it highly even to those not actively involved in endoscopic sinus surgery. I have enjoyed working on this venture tremendously, and would like to share my experience about nasal and sinus endoscopy. I hope this book guides the novice and stimulates the experienced endoscopist to greater heights.

Acknowledgements

I would like to thank the medical and nursing staff of the Tyrone County Hospital, Omagh for their help in my endeavor to mature this technique. A special mention must be made for the constant support and dedicated assistance that I have received from

Mr Hugh Mills, Chief Executive of Sperrin and Lakeland Management Unit, Mrs Bernie McCrory, General Services Manager and Mrs Martina Corrigan, Assistant General Services Manager and I should like to thank them with gratitude.

I acknowledge with thanks the commercial support received from Karl Storz, John Weiss of London and Richard Wolf (U.K.) Ltd.

I deeply appreciate the invaluable help of my son Anup in the preparation of this book especially with computer graphics and technical support and I would like to express my sincere thanks to him. I also would like to thank N. Patil for his technical assistance.

S.K. Kaluskar
Omagh, Northern Ireland, 1997

Contents

Chapter 1   **A Historical Overview** 1

Chapter 2   **Surgical Anatomy** 3

Chapter 3   **Endoscopic Anatomy** 9

Chapter 4   **Muco-Ciliary Concepts** 15

Chapter 5   **Office Nasal Endoscopy** 21

Chapter 6   **Sinus Imaging** 33

Chapter 7   **Medical Aspects of Sinusitis** 47

Chapter 8   **FESS Technique** 51

Chapter 9   **The Ethmoid Cavity: Post-Operative Care** 71

Chapter 10   **Headaches and Facial Pains** 75

Chapter 11   **Complications in FESS** 79

                          High Risk Areas in Endoscopic Sinus Surgery by T. Ohinishi 83

Chapter 12   **Prevention of Pitfalls in FESS** 91

Chapter 13   **FESS Data Analysis** 97

Chapter 14   **Tips for Beginners** 103

Chapter 15   **Broadening the Horizons** 107

Appendices 121

References 127

Index 129

Abbreviations

A	adhesions	MM	middle meatus
AN	agger nasi	MMA	middle meatal antrostomy
BE	bulla ethmoidales	MT	middle turbinate
CG	crista galli	MX	maxillary sinus
ET	Eustachian tube	NP	nasopharynx
ETh	ethmoids	ON	optic nerve
FE	fovea ethmoidales	OS	ostium
FR	frontal recess	P	pus
HS	hiatus semilunaris	PNS	post-natal space
IM	inferior meatus	PO	polyp
INA	inferior nasal antrostomy	S	septum
IC	internal carotid	SM	superior meatus
IT	inferior turbinate	SP	sphenoid
LP	lamina papyracea	ST	superior turbinate
LW	lateral wall	UP	uncinate process

Chapter 1

A Historical Overview

The study of the internal nasal contours dates back to early mankind, when the nose was predominantly associated with the sense of smell. The earliest record of an anatomical observation is in the papyrus of Abers and Egyptian tomb inscriptions, dated well before 1500 BC. This ancient culture used the nose as a route for extracting the contents of the cranial vault as part of the mummification process, thereby avoiding any facial disfigurement. This implies an intimate knowledge of the intricate relationship between the roof of the ethmoids and the brain.

The first reference to a crude Arabian nasal speculum dates back to the twelfth century AD (As Sayzari). As medicine gradually advanced, more and more attempts where made to visualise this rather inaccessible region. The first modern-day nasal speculum was designed by Markusowsky. Gabriel Fallopius (1523–1562) used a nasal speculum to aid in the removal of posteriorly situated polyps. Other methods of illuminating the nasal cavity include Borel's (1620–1671) concave mirror which reflected sunlight into the nose. The sinuses were first demonstrated as a distinct anatomical feature by Johann Riolan in the seventeenth century. Czermak in Vienna coined the term "rhinoscopy" in 1859 when he examined the post-nasal space and choanae using a mirror. Even with better speculae such as Perret's valved instruments, the problem of illumination remained a major obstacle. Up to the middle of the last century it was usually the otologist who carried out nasal examination. In 1869 Wertheim designed a small tube with an apertured mirror set at 45° at one end ("conchoscope"); he used it routinely to visualise the anterior and mid-third of the nasal cavity. However, it was not until the introduction of the fenestrated head mirror in the latter half of the nineteenth century that the other regions of the nose were made more visible. The speculae we use today owe their origins to masters of the eighteenth century such as Sir St Clair Thomson

(1859–1943), Gustav Killian (1862–1921) and Johann Thudicum (1829–1901).

Endoscopic nasal surgery has its roots both in intranasal procedures performed in the mid-nineteenth century as well as diagnostic sinoscopy which was relatively new at that time. The antral cavity was first accessed by von Mikulicz, who reported opening it through the middle meatus in 1886. Claoue published a 10-year survey of his antrostomies in 1912. The turbinates proved a major obstacle to adequate visualisation of the antrostomy site, but this was overcome by Dahmer (1909) who created a large inferior meatal antrostomy by resecting the anterior end of the inferior turbinate. He denuded the antral mucosa from the floor of the sinus, and claimed this resulted in a pain-free irrigation, often performed by the patient himself.

Claoue's survey suggests that other European rhinologists such as Boenninghaus and Hajek, who had accepted the method of wide inferior meatal antrostomy, with or without resection of the head of the inferior turbinate, were pleased with the almost immediate improvement in symptoms, especially the drying up of tenacious secretions. Lothrop in the USA (1897) carried out a wide inferior meatal antrostomy too, but he regarded this merely as an entry point for irrigation to control the infection, and inspection of the cavity.

As nasal surgeons became more aware of sinus pathophysiology, the concept of a middle meatal antrostomy was born. First described by Siebenmann in 1899, the procedure was once again aimed at giving the patient a method of irrigating his own sinuses over time. In addition, Siebenmann advocated resection of the head of the middle turbinate, and breaching the membranous fontanelle digitally. By this time, the delayed complications of inferior meatal windows were becoming apparent, as more and more surgeons reported closure and secondary problems. It is of

1

interest that Zuckerkandl in 1882 stated that this window generally remained fully patent. Caldwell (1893) emphasised the importance of the anterior ethmoid cells as the primary focus of sinus disease, and not the frontal and maxillary sinuses. Kubo in 1912 preferred a middle meatal antrostomy, and Onodi designed a perforator for this purpose around the turn of the century.

Simultaneously with the advent of middle meatal antrostomies came various photographic and other studies on muco-ciliary clearance of the cavity itself. Hilding (1931) first exhibited that carbon particles bypassed an inferior meatal antrostomy, and could leave the antral cavity and re-enter it again via an accessory ostium before finally leaving through the natural os. Proetz (1941) added information about this phenomenon, while Messerklinger provided photographic documentation demonstrating this process in the 1980s, and elucidated the concepts of muco-ciliary clearance as we know them today.

Further procedures on the lateral wall of the nose included Killian's technique of resection of the uncinate process with widening of the neighbouring ostium in 1900. The foundations of endoscopic sinus clearance, such as creating a single ethmoid volume, problems of exenteration of the most anterior cells, the risks of blind dissection, the use of local decongestants and of special curved instruments, were all expounded by Halle in 1906. The risk of middle turbinate avulsion has been described by several authors such as Davison (1969), Freedman and Kern (1979) and Dixon (1983), who mention symptoms of dryness because the nasal cavity tends to become too large.

With the advent of nasal endoscopy, the intimate relations of the sinus openings assumed even greater importance; it is in this period that sinus surgery was elevated to "watchmaker" status. Today, it is as much an art as it is a science.

Chapter 2

Surgical Anatomy

Introduction

Being a focal facial feature, the nose inspired several quaint notions, it was even considered to be an exit for bad spirits from the body! The foundation for a scientific assessment of this organ was laid down by Emil Zuckerkandl of Austria who, not without a pinch of humour, in his treatise quips "you have to suffer and tolerate a lot on this earth, even if you are only a pneumatised cavity!". In 1882 his first book, a comparative anatomy, was published, and his illustrations were so accurate that they spawned interest all over the globe. He is credited with having given rhinology the pride of place it deserves. Along the road of discovery one finds monuments to masters such as Grunwald, Onodi and Hajek. Hand in hand with these advances came innovations in histology, local anaesthesia and radiology, leading to a burst of anatomical information, reflected today in our current state-of-the-art environment of multi-angled endoscopes, computed tomography (CT), magnetic resonance imaging (MRI) and even three-dimensional scanning.

Developmental Anatomy

The basic functions of the nose include respiration; humidification, filtration and temperature control of inspired air; protection via the muco-ciliary mechanism and lysozymes; and olfaction (the paranasal sinuses probably participate in some of these). Embryologically speaking, the nose begins as olfactory placodes in the fifth week of intra-uterine life on the ventral surfaces of the fronto-nasal process. These soon become depressed to form olfactory pits, which divide the fronto-nasal process into two parts: the medial and lateral nasal processes. These form the precursors of the nasal structure.

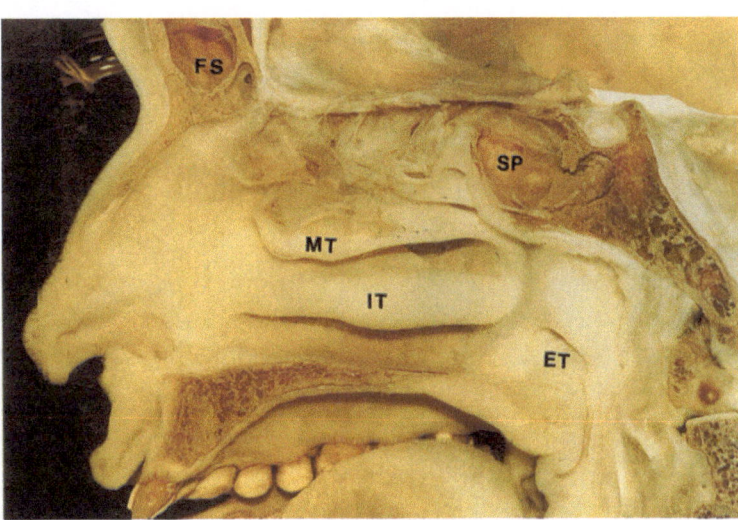

Fig. 2.1. The lateral wall of the nose showing the inferior turbinate (IT), middle turbinate (MT) and eustachian tube opening (ET). The sphenoid (SP) and frontal (FS) sinuses are also seen.

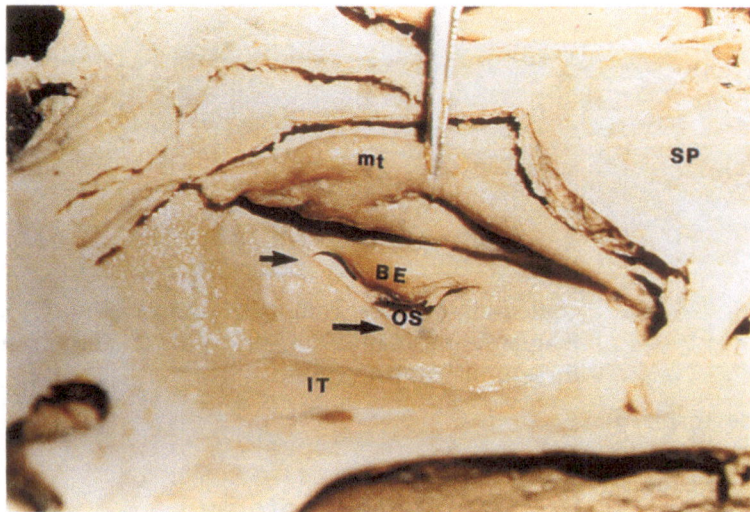

Fig. 2.2. On lifting the middle turbinate, the middle meatus comes into view. The short arrow points to the uncinate process, while the bulla ethmoidales (BE) and the natural os (OS) are also indicated.

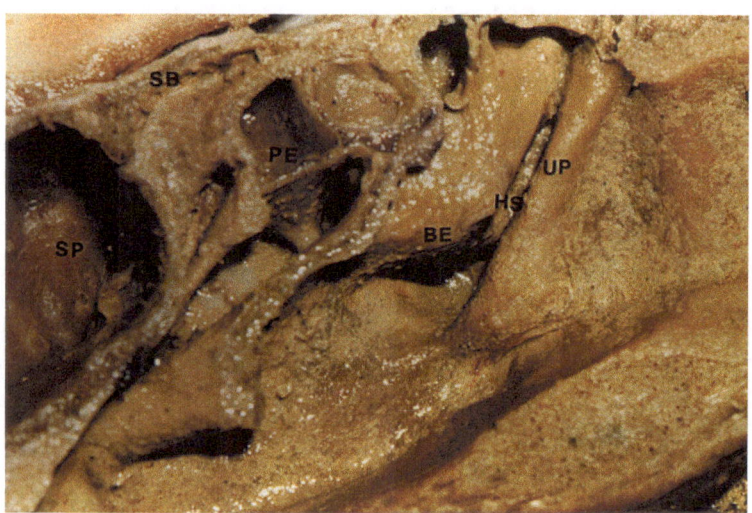

Fig. 2.3. The middle turbinate has been resected to expose the hiatus semilunaris (HS), flanked by the uncinate process (UP) and the bulla ethmoidales (BE) The posterior ethmoidal cells (PE) and sphenoidal sinus (SP) are also seen. SB, skull base.

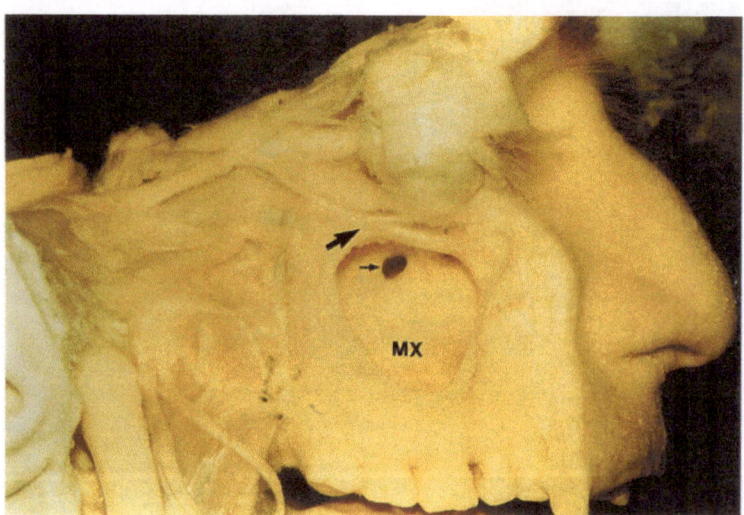

Fig. 2.4. Dissection of the maxillary sinus to show the natural os in relation to the inferior wall of the orbit. Small arrow, maxillary os; large arrow, infra-orbital nerve.

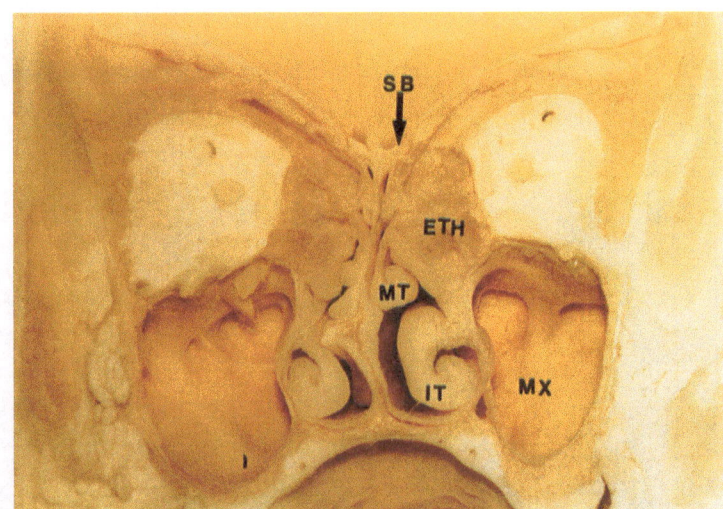

Fig. 2.5. Coronal section of the paranasal sinuses showing the maxillary sinus (MX), inferior turbinate (IT), middle turbinate (MT), ethmoid labyrinth (ETH) and the skull base (SB).

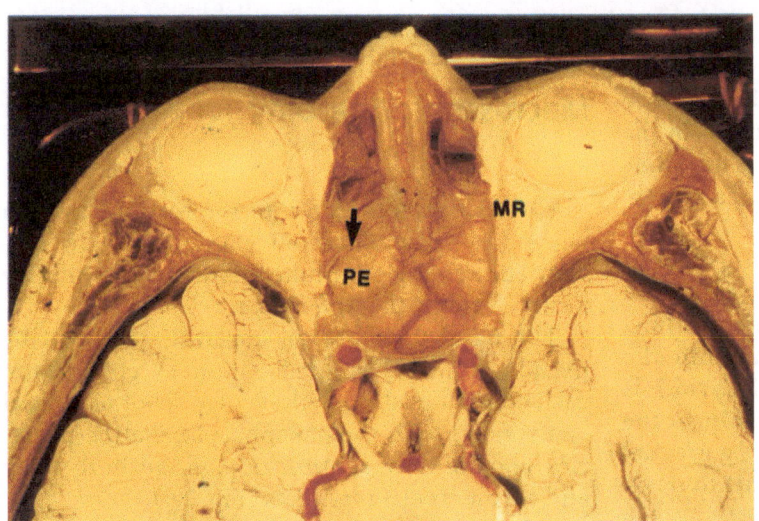

Fig. 2.6. Axial view of the ethmoid labyrinth, showing its relation to the medial rectus (MR). The internal carotid artery and optic nerves are seen to be in close proximity to the posterior-most ethmoidal cells. Arrow points to ground lamella. PE, posterior ethmoids.

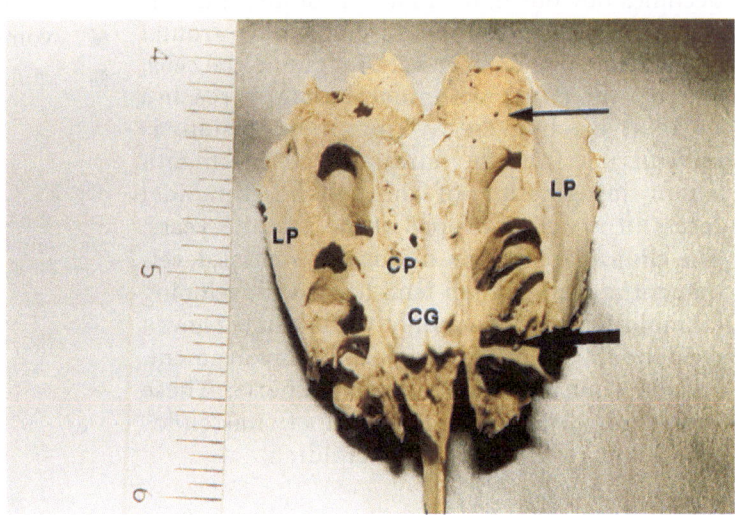

Fig. 2.7. The ethmoid bone showing the crista galli (CG), lamina papyracea (LP) and the cribriform plate (CP). Anterior (thick arrow) and posterior (thin arrow) ethmoidal cells are seen.

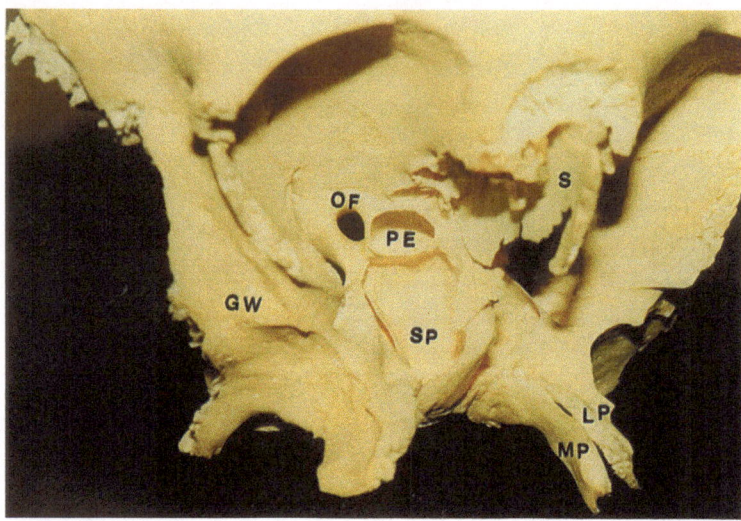

Fig. 2.8. Articluated frontal and sphenoid bones showing posterior ethmoidal cells (PE), their relation to the optic foramen (OF) and the sphenoid sinus (SP). Note that the sphenoid is not a continuation of the posterior ethmoid, but is infero-medial to it. GW, greater wing of sphenoid; S septum; MP, medial pterygoid plate; LP, lateral pterygoid plate

The maxillary sinus is seen as a shallow groove extending laterally from the infundibulum in the fourth month of intra-uterine life. The sinus begins to encroach into the maxilla at birth. Pneumatisation drives the floor of the sinus downwards until it approaches the nasal floor at the age of 8 years. The ethmoids originate from pre-formed furrows at around the same time, with the ethnoidal cells invaginating into the lateral ethmoid masses. The ethmoid labyrinth is seen to be well pneumatised at birth. Up to the age of 6 years the maxillary sinus shows a gradual growth curve, after which there is a spurt to reach its adult size by puberty.

The frontal sinus is absent at birth, and becomes obvious in the first year of life. It develops by direct extension of the whole frontal recess, from one or more anterior ethmoidal cells, or from the ethmoidal infundibulum. It reaches its adult size by puberty. The sphenoid sinus is recognisable from the third intra-uterine month as an invagination of the spheno-ethmoidal recess. It is well developed at the age of 8 years. The clinical application of this differential development is that children tend towards developing ethmoiditis more commonly, while adults show a preponderance of maxillary sinus involvement. Frontal sinusitis is rare before puberty. These facts have direct bearing on functional endoscopic sinus surgery (FESS) in children.

Macroscopic Anatomy

The anterior nares lead into the vestibule, which is lined by skin, sebaceous glands and hair follicles. The vestibule is limited above and behind by a curved ridge, the limen nasi.

The nasal passages, in contrast, are lined by pseudo-stratified ciliated columnar epithelium, each communicating with its own set of paranasal sinuses and with the nasopharynx via the posterior choana. The septum is made of both bony and cartilaginous segments (Fig. 2.9):

- perpendicular plate of ethmoid (above and behind, bony)
- vomer (below and behind, bony)
- quadrilateral cartilage (cartilaginous)

Fig. 2.9. C, cartilaginous septum; V, vomer; E, perpendicular plate of the ethmoid bone.

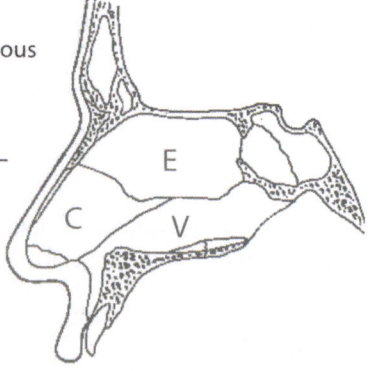

The lateral wall of the nose is its most important surface in terms of nasal dynamics. It consists of:

- medial wall of maxilla
- lateral portions of the ethmoid and lacrimal bones
- ascending process of maxilla/perpendicular plate of palatine/ medial pterygoid process

Average turbinal lengths in the adult	
Superior	7–25 mm, average 16.2 mms
Middle	30–50 mm, average 40 mms
Inferior	36–56 mm, average 46 mms

It bears three turbinates (superior, middle and inferior) overhanging their meati (occasionally a fourth "supreme" turbinate may be seen). Drainage of the paranasal sinuses occurs via ostia in the lateral wall of nose. The superior meatus bears the opening of the posterior ethmoidal cells, while the sphenoidal ostium opens into its own groove, the spheno-ethmoidal recess. The middle meatus is the most significant area of the lateral surface in this regard; it contains the openings of the anterior/middle ethmoids and the frontal sinuses. Into the anterior part of the middle meatus open the anterior ethmoid sinuses. In 50% of cases the frontal sinus opening is seen to coalesce with these openings. Into the posterior part opens the maxillary sinus. The middle ethmoidal cells have variable sites of opening, ranging from onto the bulla to above the bulla or near it. The inferior meatus receives the opening of the nasolacrimal duct. The paranasal sinus complex constitutes an intricate labyrinth of air spaces within the bones – four to each side. They are as follows:

- The *maxillary sinus* (antrum of Highmore): pyramidal in shape, its apex extends into the zygomatic process of the maxilla. It has a capacity of approximately 30 ml, thus making it the largest cavity. Its roof is the thin floor of the orbit, which is grooved by the infra-orbital nerve. The base is the alveolar process and the hard palate. In the child, this lies at the level of, or just above, the nasal floor, while it drops to 1 cm below this level in the adult. The main ostium of the sinus is situ-

ated high up between the roof and medial wall. It opens into the hiatus semilunaris in its lower part.

The maxillary sinus (usually symmetrical bilaterally)	
Length	38.5 mm
Width	26.4 mm

- The *ethmoid cells* number 8-15. Predominantly occupying the mass of the ethmoid bone, they may "invade" the agger nasi and middle turbinate, and sometimes the surrounding bones such as the maxillary, frontal and sphenoid. They may be differentiated into anterior and posterior groups, separated by a ground lamella. The anterior cells are small, and open into the upper part of the hiatus semilunaris. The posterior cells are larger, and open into the superior meatus. The ethmoid labyrinth is related to the anterior cranial fossa, the orbit, lacrimal sac and optic nerve. The anterior and posterior ethmoidal vessels and nerves pass from the orbit along the roof into the nasal fossa.

- The frontal sinus is an extended anterior ethmoidal cell. It is of variable capacity, the right and left sinuses often being asymmetrically divided by one or many septae. Each sinus drains into the infundibulum of the ethmoid via the frontal recess, which opens into its antero-superior aspect. This area is identified as the frontal recess, and is in close anatomic proximity to the frontal sinus itself. The frontal recess is not a "duct" in the true sense of the word, and hence should not be referred to as such.

- The sphenoid sinus lies behind the upper part of the nasal fossa, and occupies the body, and sometimes the wings and pterygoid processes of the sphenoid. The sinus is related to the cavernous sinus, pituitary gland, optic chiasma, olfactory tract and frontal lobe. The vidian nerve runs below its floor. In its upper part, it measures approximately 14 mm from anterior to posterior wall.

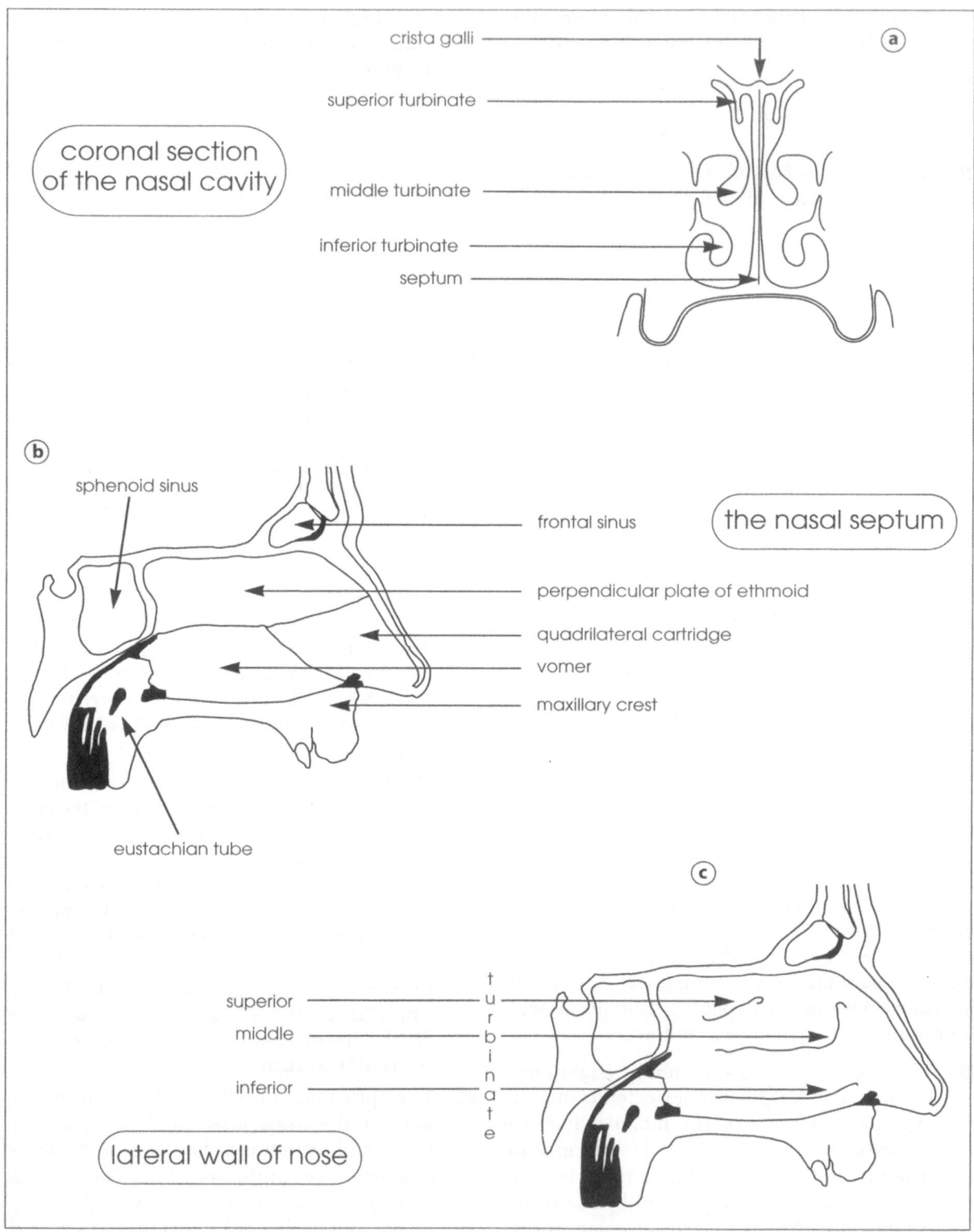

crista galli

superior turbinate

coronal section of the nasal cavity

middle turbinate

inferior turbinate

septum

sphenoid sinus

the nasal septum

frontal sinus

perpendicular plate of ethmoid

quadrilateral cartridge

vomer

maxillary crest

eustachian tube

superior

middle

inferior

turbinate

lateral wall of nose

Fig. 2.10a–c. Various anatomical structures of the nasal cavity. **a** coronal section; **b** nasal septum; **c** lateral wall of the nose.

Chapter 3

Endoscopic Anatomy

Anatomy is often a matter of perspective, and this truism is apt as never before when applied to the nose and paranasal sinuses. Macroscopic descriptions found in most standard textbooks often do not correlate to the straight or angled endoscopic view the surgeon has to rely on when traversing these landscapes. He must develop a feel for volume as he looks at area, and must be able to build up a three-dimensional map allowing him to know exactly where he is, where the openings and the danger zones lie, and what structures are closely related. We present the anatomy of this complex region as a series of building blocks, to be put together and further enhanced by CT scanning. Extensive photographic documentation of endoscopic anatomy and pathological findings is to be found in chapter 5.

An endoscopic view of the lateral wall of nose shows:

- ostio-meatal complex
- turbinates
- fontanelles
- agger nasi cells

Ostio-meatal complex

The ostio-meatal complex (anterior to posterior) consists of:

- middle meatus
- uncinate process
- hiatus semilunaris
- infundibulum
- maxillary ostium
- bulla ethmoidales

Middle Meatus

The middle meatus is the space underneath the middle turbinate, in which lies the hiatus semilunaris, along with some of the paranasal sinus openings. It also contains parts of the fontanelles

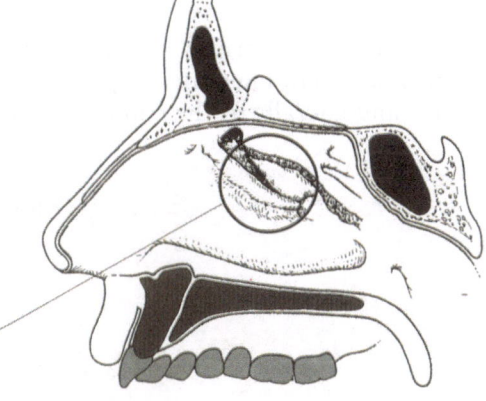

Fig. 3.1. Ostio-meatal complex (OMC). MT, middle turbinate; BE, bulla ethmoides; UP, uncinate process; arrow shows ostium.

and the bulla ethmoidales (middle ethmoidal cells). Anteriorly is the opening of the frontal sinus along with the anterior ethmoidal cells. The posterior portion bears the opening of the maxillary sinus, and may contain an accessory opening in 10%–40% of patients. It is important to note that the fronto-nasal "duct" is more a recess into which the frontal sinus opens, and should be called as such.

As Caldwell emphasised in 1893, "in the diagnosis ... beyond dispute the one absolute proof is the detection of pus escaping from the sinus. This may be secured in all the cells without resorting to exploratory operations ... the relative positions of the sinus openings is of diagnostic value".

Uncinate Process

The uncinate process (from the Latin *uncinatus* meaning hooked) is a part of the ethmoid bone, about 7–22 mm in length. It forms a constant curved landmark on the lateral wall of the nose, and runs from above downwards and from the front backwards. It is of crucial importance to the endoscopic surgeon as he prepares to access the infundibulum, of which it forms the antero-medial boundary. Its sharp, cephalic border forms the margin of the hiatus semilunaris.

Hiatus Semilunaris

The hiatus semilunaris is a 1–2 mm wide two-dimensional cleft, lined medially by the uncinate process and laterally by the ethmoidal infundibulum. In its anterior part lie the openings of the anterior ethmoidal cells and the frontal recess, while the lower and posterior part contains the natural opening of the maxillary sinus. The posterior relation is to the bulla ethmoidales.

Infundibulum

Mosher in 1929 described the infundibulum as the "uncinate groove" (a term which has not stood the test of time), while Myerson (1932) called it "a channel between the ethmoid bulla and the uncinate process". It is a three dimensional space, and is, in fact, a meeting point for drainage of the frontal, anterior/middle ethmoidal and maxillary sinuses. It belongs to the anterior ethmoids. The medial wall is constituted by the entire length of the uncinate process enveloped in its mucosa. The lateral wall is largely provided by the medial orbital wall, while the frontal process of the maxilla and, in some cases, the lacrimal bone makes up the remainder. At times, the infundibulum may end as a blind recess anteriorly, depending upon the position of the uncinate process in its upper part. The posterior boundary of the ethmoidal infundibulum is largely the anterior surface of the bulla ethmoidales, from where the infundibulum opens into the middle meatus, through the hiatus semilunaris.

From the surgical point of view, it is important to remember that the ethmoidal infundibulum may be quite shallow when the uncinate process is in close proximity to the lamina papyracea. Sometimes in the presence of paradoxical turbinate and/or concha bullosa the ethmoidal

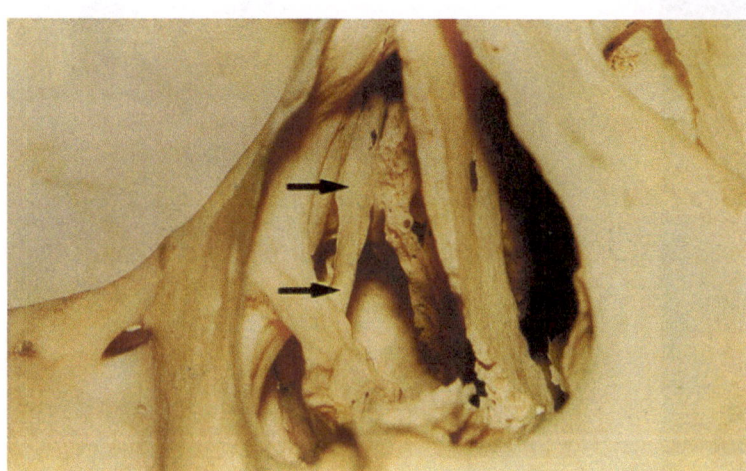

Fig. 3.2. A dissected bony specimen shows the uncinate process of the ethmoid bone (arrows) as a curved projection forming the medial wall of the ethmoidal infundibulum.

infundibulum may be completely obliterated, thus resulting in recurrent sinus infections.

Maxillary Ostium (antro-nasal channel)

This is not merely an opening into the lateral wall of the nose; rather it is a channel for communication between the infundibulum and the maxillary sinus. It is at the junction of the medial maxillary wall and the floor of the orbit, halfway between the anterior and posterior maxillary walls (approximately 2 cm from each). It is normally horizontal or oblique. It has two orifices, nasal and antral, which can differ in size, shape and direction. Looking out of the sinus at the ostium, one might see the uncinate process anterosuperiorly, and the bulla ethmoidales posteroinferiorly. Accessory ostia may be seen in 10%–40% of patients.

Bulla Ethmoidales

The bulla ethmoidales is a large middle ethmoidal cell with thin delicate walls, often with its own opening. Sited just posteriorly to the hiatus semilunaris, it also forms the posterior boundary of the maxillary ostium. It opens into the ethmoid infundibulum or into the sinus lateralis. Sometimes there is a distinct furrow along its medial wall. Sometimes the bulla may extend to

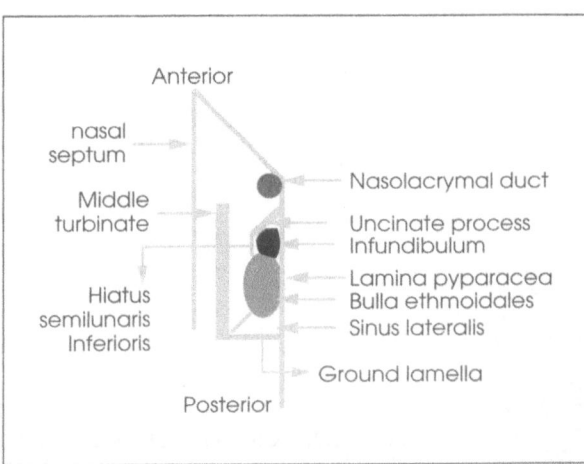

Fig. 3.3. Schematic diagram of the right ethmoidal infundibulum.

atttach to the vertical portion of the ground lamella, and/or the roof of the ethmoid. When it fuses with the roof of the ethmoid, the interveing space between it and the ground lamella is termed sinus lateralis. A very large bulla may obliterate this space, in which case the posterior wall of the bulla becomes the anterior surface of the ground lamella (see Fig. 3.3).

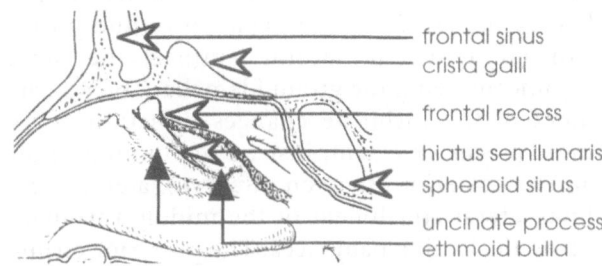

Fig. 3.4. Lateral wall of the nose.

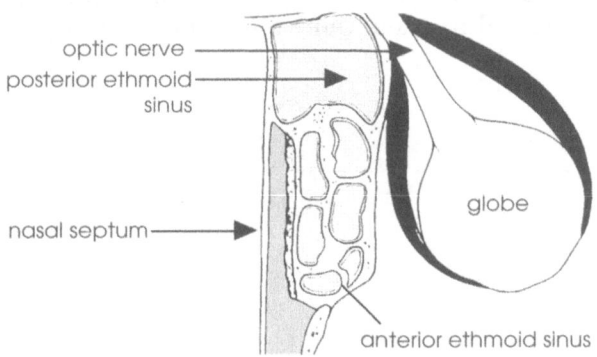

Fig. 3.5. Axial view of the ethmoids and orbit.

Turbinates

The three most important features on the lateral wall of the nose are the inferior, middle and superior turbinates with their meati (a fourth "supreme" turbinate may sometimes be seen). The supreme, superior and middle turbinates are an integral part of the ethmoid labyrinth, whereas the inferior turbinate is a separate bone. All the turbinates conceal their meati, into which open the paranasal sinuses.

A centimetre behind the anterior end of the inferior turbinate is the opening of the naso-lacrimal duct into the inferior meatus, often recognised by a surrounding crescent of mucosal fold. Gentle massage of the lacrimal sac often causes exudation of a tear-drop into the inferior meatus.

The middle turbinate is by far the most crucial landmark for the endoscopist. It has two attachments: an anterior one extending superiorly to articulate with the cribriform plate of the ethmoid bone; and the more important attachment to the lamina papyracea separating anterior and posterior ethmoids via several laminae, the most significant being the ground lamella. The attachment of the turbinate changes direction at its most posterior extent; instead of running in an antero-posterior direction, it curves laterally, the final lateral attachment of the middle turbinate being the lamina papyracea. The posterior termination of the middle turbinate lies along the frontal or coronal plane, and is called the basal or ground lamella. Behind this one finds a few large posterior ethmoidal cells, into which juts the sphenoid rostrum. Quite often, the anterior part

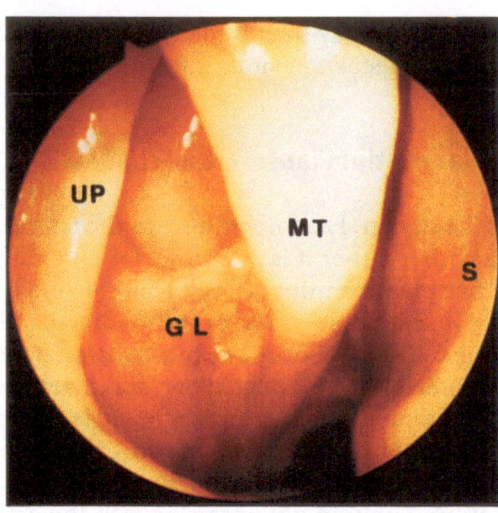

Fig. 3.6. Endoscopic view of the right middle meatus showing the ground lamella. UP, uncinate process; gl, ground lamella; MT, middle turbinate; s, septum.

of the middle turbinate contains an air space (conchal sinus) which may become infected in keeping with generalised inflammation of the ethmoid labyrinth.

Into the middle meatus open the frontal sinus and anterior/middle ethmoidal cells (anteriorly) and the maxillary sinus (posteriorly). The posterior ethmoidal sinuses open into the superior meatus, and the sphenoidal opening is into the spheno-ethmoidal recess situated postero-superiorly to the superior turbinate.

Important endoscopic measurements from the anterior nasal spine	
uncinate process	5.2 cms
anterior wall of sphenoid	6.1 cms
sphenoidal lumen	7.3 cms

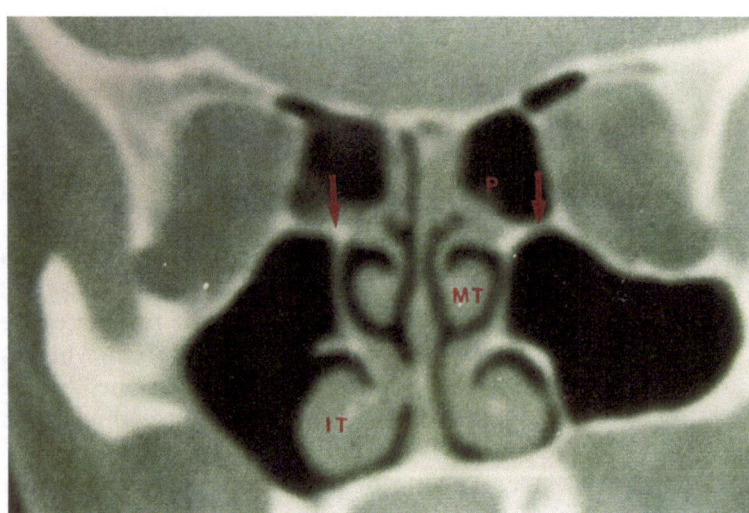

Fig. 3.7. Coronal CT scan view showing the ground lamellae on both sides (arrows). IT, inferior turbinate; MT, middle turbinate; P, posterior ethmoids.

Fontanelles

These are fibrous membranes stretched across the medial wall of the maxillary sinus. They are divided into anterior and posterior mainly by the uncinate process and the conchal process of the inferior concha. The accessory sinus openings are to be found in these membranes. In fact, if one or more openings on the lateral wall of the nose are seen on nasal endoscopy, they are always accessory ostia, and *not* the natural ostium of the maxillary sinus. Also, antro-choanal polyps exit the sinus through an accessory opening.

Agger Nasi Cells

These are the anterior-most ethmoidal cells, and form an intimate relation with the frontal recess. They lie just anterior to the superior attachment of the middle turbinate, and anterior to the frontal recess. These cells can dissect the lacrimal bone or the ascending process of the maxilla. Owing to their proximity to the frontal recess, it is wise to open these cells to access the frontal recess if there is any disease in the frontal sinus. Disease in this region may block the infundibulum and thereby the frontal recess. *A significant number of failed FESS procedures are due to inadequate clearance of this area.* Endoscopically, one often recognises these cells by a characteristic bulge on the lateral wall of the nose near the lateral attachment of the middle turbinate.

Chapter 4

Muco-Ciliary Concepts

Introduction

Unfortunately, the nose, with its convoluted internal architecture, is prone to obstructive disease. Although the muco-ciliary pathways work harmoniously in health, infection can rapidly throw this delicate mechanism into disarray. Most infections of the paranasal sinuses arise from a primary focus in the nose. Logically, therefore, recurrent disease implies an occult focus. The infection may also be secondary to trauma, of dental origin, or may occur via the blood stream. The key area of the lateral wall of the nose, the ostio-meatal complex, is most affected, thus blocking the openings of the maxillary and frontal sinuses. The most important site to be affected is the anterior ethmoidal complex, as the frontal and maxillary sinuses are dependent on them for their drainage. Messerklinger's work spanning over two decades established the genetically predetermined pathways of muco-ciliary clearance within the paranasal sinus system.

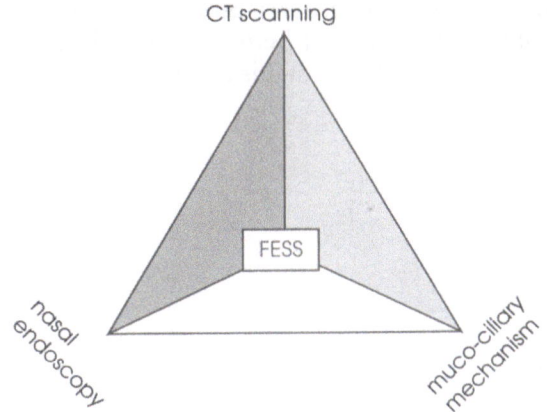

Fig. 4.1. The three factors fundamental to the concept of functional endoscopic sinus surgery (FESS).

Predisposing factors such as high septal deviations and/or spurs, medial/lateral rotation of the uncinate process, middle turbinate abnormalities such as knobbing, paradoxicity and conchosity go hand-in-hand with inflammatory and/or allergic processes to give rise to a vicious cycle of impaired ventilation and drainage of the sinuses. This knowledge, along with advances in imaging techniques and multi-angled endoscopic evaluation, led to the concept of FESS as it is known today.

Muco-Ciliary Clearance in the Nose and Paranasal Sinuses

General

Transport at a cellular level is integral to life itself. The movement of ions across cell membranes, the excretion of wastes from organs and the passage of nutrients all contribute to harmony and balance.

The nose, a point of entry for both air and foreign particles, relies on a very intricate system of muco-ciliary clearance (MCC) for its well-being. Two phylogenetically ancient systems blend to provide for this phenomenon: the production of mucus, which is present even in primitive algae, and the principle of ciliary locomotion, seen in certain protozoa.

Historical Aspects

The story of ciliary function investigation began in 1677, when Johannes Ham, a student of Leiden, first observed ciliary movements under a microscope. This was later confirmed by Van Leeuwenhoeck in seminal fluid. It took over a century, however, for Purkinje and Valentin to correlate this movement with the continuous cleansing action of ciliated epithelium. Martius in 1884 demonstrated ciliary motion stroboscopically and computed the beat frequency. The early half of the twentieth century saw a number of studies being carried out by pioneers in the field: Antweiler, Messerklinger, Negus and Proetz among others. Coloured particles and dyes (Hilding 1931, Tremble 1948, Evert 1965), and radioactive substances (Proctor and Wagner 1965) have all been introduced into the nasal cavity as markers for ciliary speed. Hilding successfully calculated the energy of ciliary epithelium in hen trachea. His contribution to animal and clinical studies has been monumental.

The introduction of the electron microscope provided new impetus to the investigation of ciliary phenomena. Jakus and Hall (1946) were responsible for demonstrating the longitudinal fibrillae within a single cilium. Further details were provided by Fawcett and Porter in 1954.

The relationship between nasal dysfunction and impaired mucociliary clearance has been described by Quinlan (1969), Puchelle (1981) and Sakakura (1985). Recurrent assaults on the lining of the nose lead to oedema and obstruction of the sinus openings, thus lowering intra-luminal oxygen tension, and encouraging the growth of anaerobic organisms. Exotoxin release then acts to further impede ciliary movement, this setting up a vicious cycle within the sinus. The aim of FESS is to re-establish normal drainage and ventilation channels by creating an easily accessible cavity. This encourages the muco-ciliary mechanism to regain harmonious function. Hence this form of surgery is known as "functional".

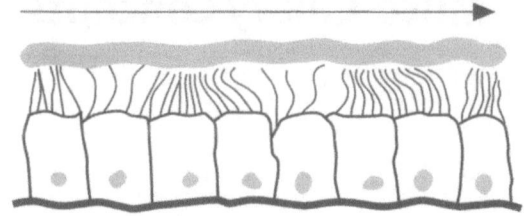

ciliated cells propelling thr overlying mucous blanket

Fig. 4.2. Ciliated cells propelling the overlying mucous blanket.

Cilia

Phylogenetically, cilia are found in all animal species, including the nematodes. In the vertebrates, they are important in respiratory function, as well as the movement of spermatozoa and fallopian tube transport. Individual cilia move in a whip-like fashion, thus providing a lateral force to the overlying substance. When viewed in conjunction with their neighbours, this movement converts to one of continuous, wave-like motion.

The extent of ciliary epithelium in the airways is not constant, and is defined by environmental and genetic factors. A single ciliated epithelium cell carries between 50 and 300 cilia on its surface. The length of cilia in vertebrates is 3–8 µm, the diameter being 0.1–0.3 µm, with a narrowing towards the tip. The shaft contains nine peripheral tubules and two central single tubules. Energy for ciliary movement is ATP driven, and the average beat frequency is 5–20 Hz at 37 °C. Cilia are upright and rigid during the beat, and curved during the recovery phase. Mucus consists of 98% water, the rest being composed of albumin, globulin, glycoproteins and salts.

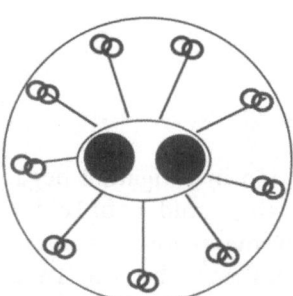

Fig. 4.3. Each cilium consists of the nine double microtubules surrounding two central microtubules.

All in all, MCC depends on an intact, metachronously beating ciliary epithelium, and an accurately balanced mucus layer of optimal viscoelasticity. Its physical properties thus seem to be more important than its biochemical properties.

MCC of the nose and paranasal sinuses is a highly directional activity. It is independent of body position, and is mainly directed backwards into the nasopharynx, except for a very small amount of forward movement at the very anterior end of the nasal septum. Within the maxillary antrum, MCC follows a star shaped pattern, originating from the floor and ascending into a spiral to end at the natural os. *Even in the presence of an inferior antrostomy opening, mucus still moves towards the natural ostium.* Messerklinger (1978) has shown that ethmoid and sphenoid clearance is directly through their respective ostia, whereas the frontal sinus shows circular traffic, only a small part of which exits via the fronto-nasal recess into the nose. Hence an increase in viscosity leads to almost immediate stasis in the frontal sinus.

Factors Influencing Mucociliary Clearance

Various parameters such as temperature and humidity affect MCC; the earliest studies in this regard are those of Engelmann (1877) and Dixon et al. (1905). Engelmann found increasing activity up to 45 °C, followed by a rapid decline. The optimal beat frequency lay between 30 and 40 °C. However, Proetz (1941) has stated that "the only natural enemy to cilia is excessive drying". Optimal relative humidity is around 90%. Neutral pH values are associated with good ciliary activity. Ciliary stasis rapidly sets in outside pH values of 7–10. Similarly, correct osmolarity and oxygen tension are essential for ciliary movements. Oxygenation is maintained both by diffusion from circulating blood, as well as from the surface itself. Interestingly, a mechanical load such as blood clot or mucus plug accelerates MCC.

A wide range of drugs and chemicals affect the mucociliary clearance. Smoking is known to have a deleterious effect, while sympathomimetic decongestant nose drops have been shown to retard ciliary function.

Pathophysiology of Sinusitis

Common pathogens found in the maxillary sinus are pneumococci, *Haemophilus influenzae* and other anaerobic organisms. Quite often there is underlying damage to the epithelium as a result of viral infection, this leads to exudate formation

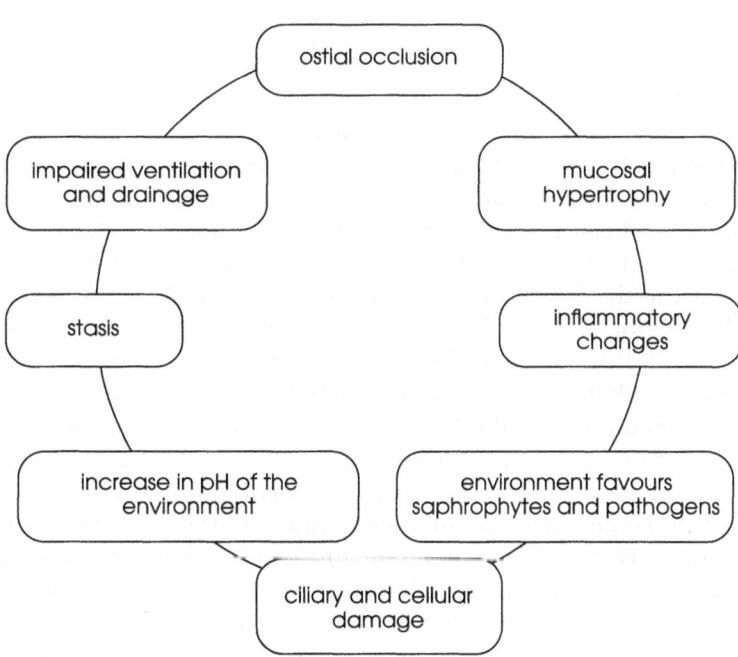

Fig. 4.4. The vicious circle of ostium closure and recurrent sinus infections.

and retention of secretions. The damaged mucosa and secretions form a favourable substrate for bacterial colonisation. As the oxygen tension in antral air is mainly dependent on the patency of the ostium and absorption by mucosa (Aust and Drettner 1974b), its closure leads to low partial pressure of oxygen PO_2 and high CO_2 levels and a rise in antral pH, thus affecting ciliary mechanisms (Aust and Drettner 1974b, Frederick and Braude 1974). Thus impaired ventilation due to ostial occlusion facilitates bacterial and cellular influence on the gas environment in such a way that heavy growth of anaerobes is initiated and maintained and a serous sinusitis is changed into a more purulent variety.

Clinical Assessment of Muco-Ciliary Function

Since Martius in 1884 used stroboscopy to study muco-ciliary function of the nose, a number of methods, both direct and indirect, have been used by other workers. Hilding in 1931 and Tremble in 1948 used dyes and coloured particles and timed their passage through the nasal cavities. Harper et al. (1962) resorted to radioactive technetium monitored by serial scanning. These methods, though sophisticated, often proved cumbersome for routine clinical use. Anderson (1974) introduced the use of saccharin placed on the nasal mucosa; by recording the time interval before the patient felt a sweet taste, an estimate of mucociliary clearance could be made. His technique has since been used by others in the field. Ginzel and Ellum (1980) and Hady (1983) modified this by using dyed saccharin in order to record dual observations.

In addition, researchers like King (1935), Flottes (1960), used an oil- or water-based contrast medium specifically to assess the mucociliary function of the maxillary sinus.

In our review of world literature we could not find a single instance of muco-ciliary studies being performed in patients of FESS using the saccharin test. Hence we undertook a prospective, controlled project involving 40 patients, and measured their "saccharin times" before and after surgery. Initially the injection technique was perfected on cadavers, and it was found that the solution could be easily instilled into the antrum via the membranous anterior fontanelle as an outpatient procedure.

Ten normal volunteers were initially chosen as a control study. Care was taken to eliminate those with nasal or sinus complaints. None of the control group suffered from any allergies.

Forty random patients with symptoms and signs of chronic sinusitis formed the test group. These patients had all suffered from chronic recurrent sinus disease (nasal obstruction, postnasal drip, headache) for over a year. Diagnosis was confirmed by office endoscopy and coronal CT scans in all cases. All findings were recorded on a computer compatible proforma.

A standardised sterile solution of 25% saccharin was employed. All patients were tested in identical environmental conditions. They were instructed not to sniff forcibly, and to swallow at frequent intervals. The nature of the test solution was not revealed to the patient, they were merely asked to indicate any unusual taste they noticed.

Pre-operative assessment was carried out 24 hours prior to surgery, while post-operative recordings were done at 1, 3 and 6 months.

The procedure was carried out in the sitting position. Pre-operative recordings required limited local anaesthesia (4% xylocaine) in the region of the anterior fontanelle. A tuberculin syringe with a No.17 needle was employed. The needle was given a slight angulation in order to access the lateral nasal wall. 0.5 ml of saccharin were instilled into the antrum via the anterior fontanelle. In postoperative cases, the middle meatal antrostomy itself was used as an entry the antrum. No complications were noted during the study.

The control group exhibited a mean clearance time of 18 minutes (ranging from 12 to 25 minutes). In the patient group, pre-operative readings averaged at 46 minutes (36–62 minutes). Post-operative results at 1, 3 and 6 months are as shown in Fig 4.9. At 6 months, the reading was 23 minutes (range 18–42 minutes). This group consisted of 32 patients, eight having been lost to follow-up.

Our results showed a marked reduction in clearance times post-operatively, which was statistically significant which corresponded well with improvement in symptom profiles. We therefore propose this technique as a simple, safe and reli-

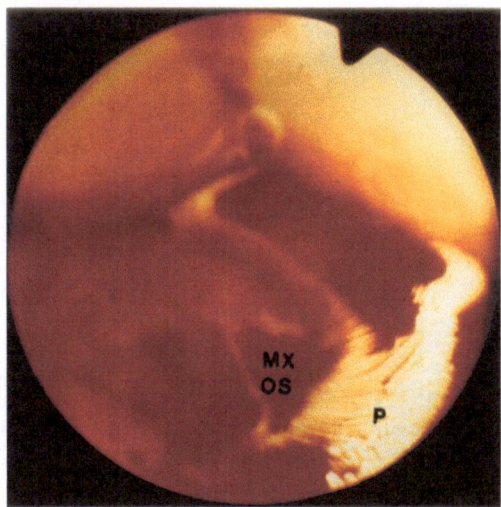

Fig. 4.5. Intra-operative picture of the left maxillary sinus showing pus (P) tracking towards the natural ostium (MX OS).

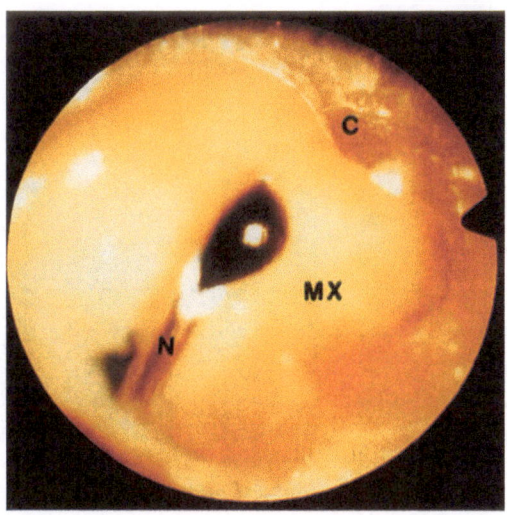

Fig. 4.7. Left maxillary antrum in the cadaver, showing instillation of a drop of dye through the anterior fontanelle. This was the first phase of our muco-ciliary clearance study (before actual patient trials). C, cannula; MX, maxillary sinus; N, needle.

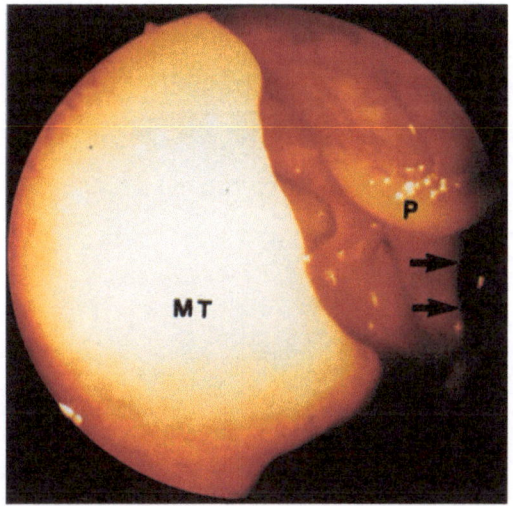

Fig. 4.6. Left-operated nasal cavity showing muco-pus (P) recirculating between a middle meatal antrostomy (arrows) and an accessory ostium. Care should be taken to remove the bridge of bone between the natural and the accessory ostium. MT, middle turbinate.

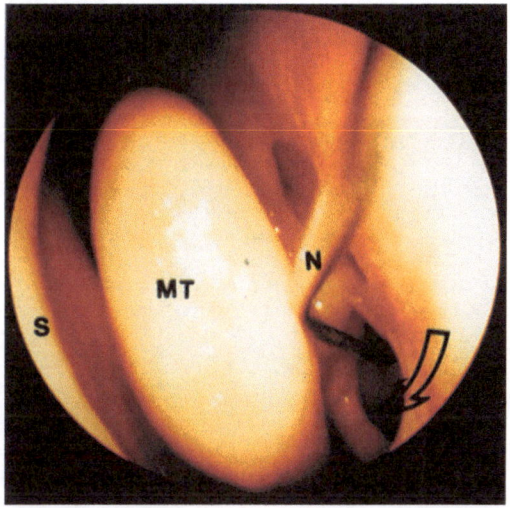

Fig. 4.8. Muco-ciliary study: patient trial. Post-operative view of the left middle meatal antrostomy (arrow) showing needle (N) being inserted into the maxillary sinus to instill standardised saccharin solution. S, septum; MT, middle turbinate.

able method of assessing results of surgery. Furthermore, the method could act as a preoperative indicator of ciliary motility disorders, as prognosis in these cases is distinctly poor.

The study shows a distinct delay in MCC time in chronic sinusitis cases as compared with controls. There is a definite improvement in these patients after FESS, almost reaching normal levels.

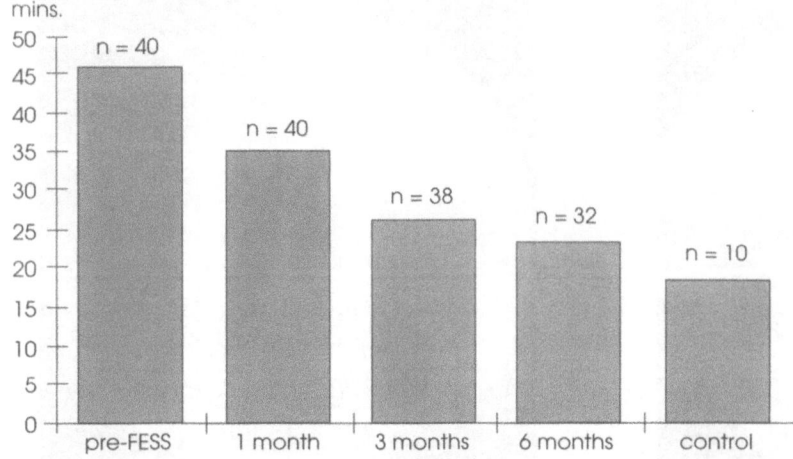

Fig. 4.9. Average clearance timings in control and pre- and post-FESS groups.

Saccharin proves to have several advantages: it is easily obtained, non-toxic and well recognised by the patient. The test itself is easily performed, reproducible, and requires no elaborate equipment.

In conclusion, as our understanding of the basic principles that control nasal and sinus function deepens, we come closer to achieving what is best for the patient. In addition to measuring MCC times, one could also focus on other parameters such as the ciliary beat frequency and electron microscope studies. Furthermore, appropriate tests are available for mucus secretion disorders such as cystic fibrosis and Young's syndrome which can also cause abnormal MCC.

Chapter 5

Office Nasal Endoscopy

Evolution of Nasal Endoscopy

It was Hirschmann in 1903 who used a modified cystoscope for diagnostic purposes in nose and sinus. Later on Reichert (1902), Valentin (1903) and Sargnon (1908) also used the endoscopic technique for the removal of foreign bodies and opening of cysts. The endoscope was inserted either through a dental socket or the anterior antral wall. Spielberg in 1922 described an alternative route to the sinuses through the inferior meatus. The scope of endoscopy in the nose and sinuses was enchanced with the introduction of better and brighter rod-based telescopes by Hopkins in the 1960s. With this development the diagnosis of nose and sinus pathologies became more precise and photographic archiving was made possible (Timm 1965, Messerklinger 1972, Draf 1973). The endoscopic evaluation of nose and sinus disease is well established across the globe. In addition to the diagnostic capabilities and surgery of the nose and sinuses the endoscope is used to perform endoscopic biopsies, to examine and irrigate the maxillary sinuses and carry out toilet post-operatively (Reynolds and Brandow 1975, Buiter 1976). Now the endoscope is used routinely for localisation of posterior epistaxis and subsequent cauterisation, excision of mucoceles, tumors of paranasal sinuses, orbital decompression and dacryocystorhinostomy(DCR).

We strongly recommend the endoscope's use even in those departments which do not routinely perform endoscopic sinus surgery, as it often reveals hidden pathologies. It is, in a sense, to sinus pathology what the microscope is to ear disease. If, for example, examination were to reveal ethmoid disease in a patient presenting with chronic sinusitis, it would be fruitless to carry out any form of surgery on the maxillary and/or frontal sinuses *per se*.

Instruments and Technique

Our routine technique uses a 4 mm, 30° Hopkins rod rigid endoscope. Although the 0° endoscope has been widely advocated for out-patient endoscopy, we would recommend its use only to the early stages of practice, when the surgeon is building up his depth perception and anatomical orientation. The very lie of the lateral wall requires an angled approach, especially when assessing the ostio-meatal complex.

The patient is examined in the sitting position. A side arm allows observation by trainee. The nose may be anaesthetised by application of cotton wicks soaked in 4% cocaine-adrenaline (care must be taken to squeeze out excess solution thoroughly to prevent absorption through the pharyngeal mucosa).

The nose is examined by three passes. The first pass traverses the floor of the nose, first examining the inferior meatus for previous antrostomy, etc. The endoscope is then guided further backwards towards the posterior choanae, examining the eustachian tube orifice, fossa of Rosenmullar and nasopharynx. Any pathology of and around the eustachian tube opening such as post-nasal discharge and mucosal oedema is noted. It is important to note that the anterior group of

First pass	
inferior meatus	? naso-lacrimal duct opening
	previous antrostomy
floor of the nose	
post-nasal space	
eustachian tube orifice	
mucus channels	

Second pass

lateral wall of nose	agger nasi
	polyps
	accesory ostia
	uncinate process
middle meatus	hiatus semilunaris
	bulla ethmoides
	natural os
	ground lamella
middle turbinate deformity	

Third pass

superior turbinate/meatus
spheno-ethmoidal recess
sphenoidal ostium

sinuses drain in front of the opening, while secretions from the posterior group pass behind it. Rotating the endoscope allows examination of the contralateral tubal opening as well as the roof of the nasopharynx. The second and most important pass examines the ostio-meatal complex. It includes a detailed assessment of the agger nasi cells , middle turbinate and high deviation of septum. The endoscope then focuses on the uncinate process, and is gently guided into the middle meatus and rotated to bring the lateral wall of the nose into view. Here most frequently seen are the hiatus semilunaris, bulla ethmoidales, rarely a nasal view of the maxillary ostium, ground lamella and various pathologies. On the lateral wall accessory ostia (punched out appearance) may be found in the fontanelles. The third pass is made between the septum and the posterior part of the middle turbinate. The endoscope is directed superiorly to examine the superior turbinate and meatus, the spheno-ethmoidal recess and the sphenoidal ostium. Findings are recorded on a computer-compatible proforma. In paediatric noses where a 4 mm endoscope may be too large and hence traumatic, we employ a 2.7 mm endoscope.

Common Findings

Agger Nasi Cells. These most anterior ethmoid cells are usually pneumatised from the frontal recess and lacrimal bone. They may obstruct the frontal recess and if infected may spread infection into the frontal sinus. They are located immediately anterior to the middle turbinate and drain into the infundibulum.

Accessory Ostium. This is present in the fontanelle (anterior or posterior) in about 10%–40% of patients. Clinically they appear as "punched-out holes". They should not be mistaken for natural ostium. The bridge of tissue between accessory os and natural os should be removed to prevent recirculation of mucus into maxillary sinus.

Uncinate Process. This varies in length from 4 to 22 mm. It is a constant curved landmark on the lateral wall forming the antero-inferior boundary of the ethmoidal infundibulum. If it is enlarged, or rotated, it blocks the infundibulum.

Paradoxical Middle Turbinate. The normal curvature of the middle turbinate is convex medially; however, if the contour is reversed, it bulges laterally and hence obstructs the middle meatus. This predisposes to narrowing of the ostio-meatal complex (OMC) leading to infection.

Concha Bullosa. This is a pneumatisation of the middle turbinate with its own opening (Zuckerkandl, 1893). Quite often it acts as a reservoir of infection for recurrent ethmoiditis and blocks the middle meatus. It may also contribute to headaches.

Polyps and Discharge. Small polyps not seen on anterior rhinoscopy can be easily seen with an endoscope and the site and flow of muco-pus in the nasal cavity is diagnostic, as observed by Caldwell in 1893.

Bulla Ethmoidales. A large ethmoidal cell in the middle meatus may obstruct the OMC thus predisposing to recurrent infection and headaches.

Septal Spur. A high deviation of septum may also contribute to narrowing of the OMC.

5.1

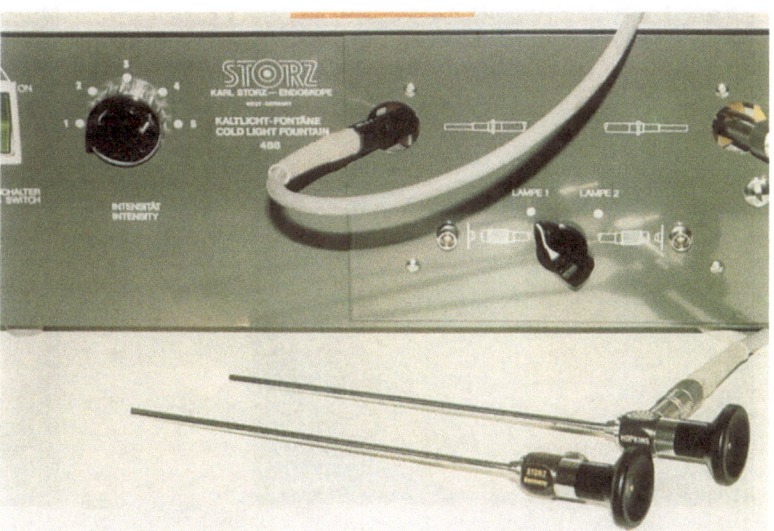

Fig. 5.1. Fibre optic light source (250 watts) with 4 mm 0° and 30° endoscopes. This wattage allows for good photographic documentation.

Fig. 5.2. The endoscope is supported by the left thumb as it enters either nostril; the remaining four fingers of the left hand fix the head.

Fig. 5.3. First pass, showing the left nare (N) and the septum (S).

Fig. 5.4. Further inwards is the inferior turbinate (IT), the middle turbinate (MT) is seen in the distance. This is roughly the view one would obtain by anterior rhinoscopy. S, septum.

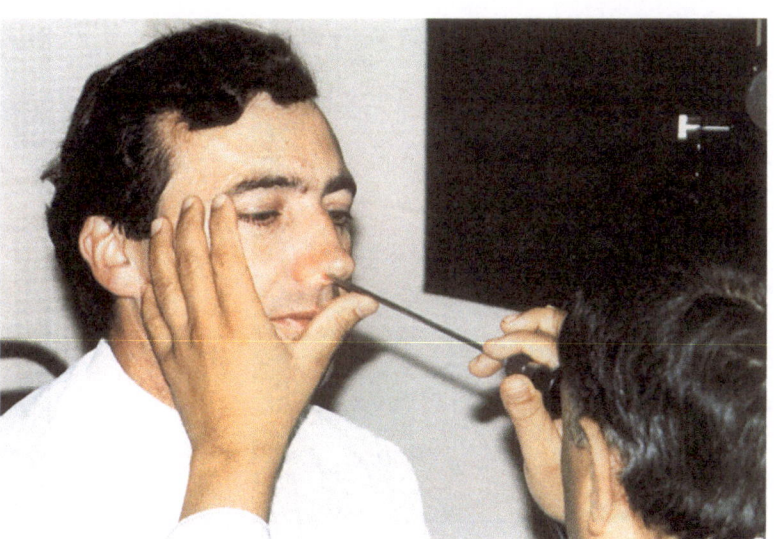

5.2

5.3

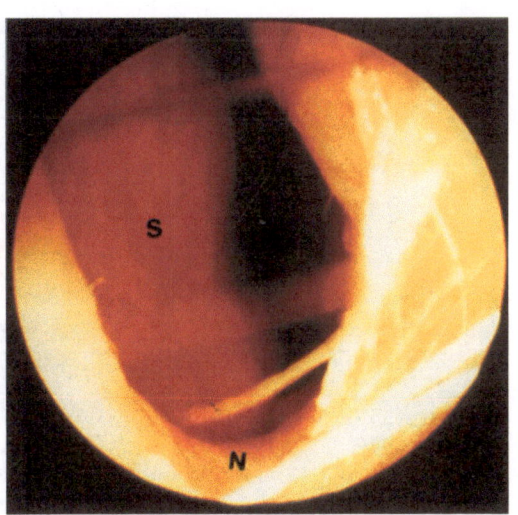

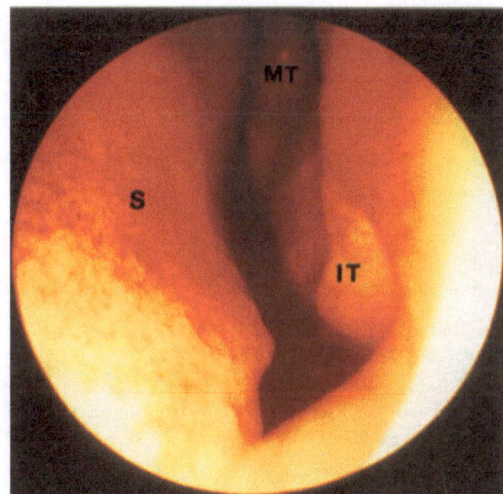

5.4

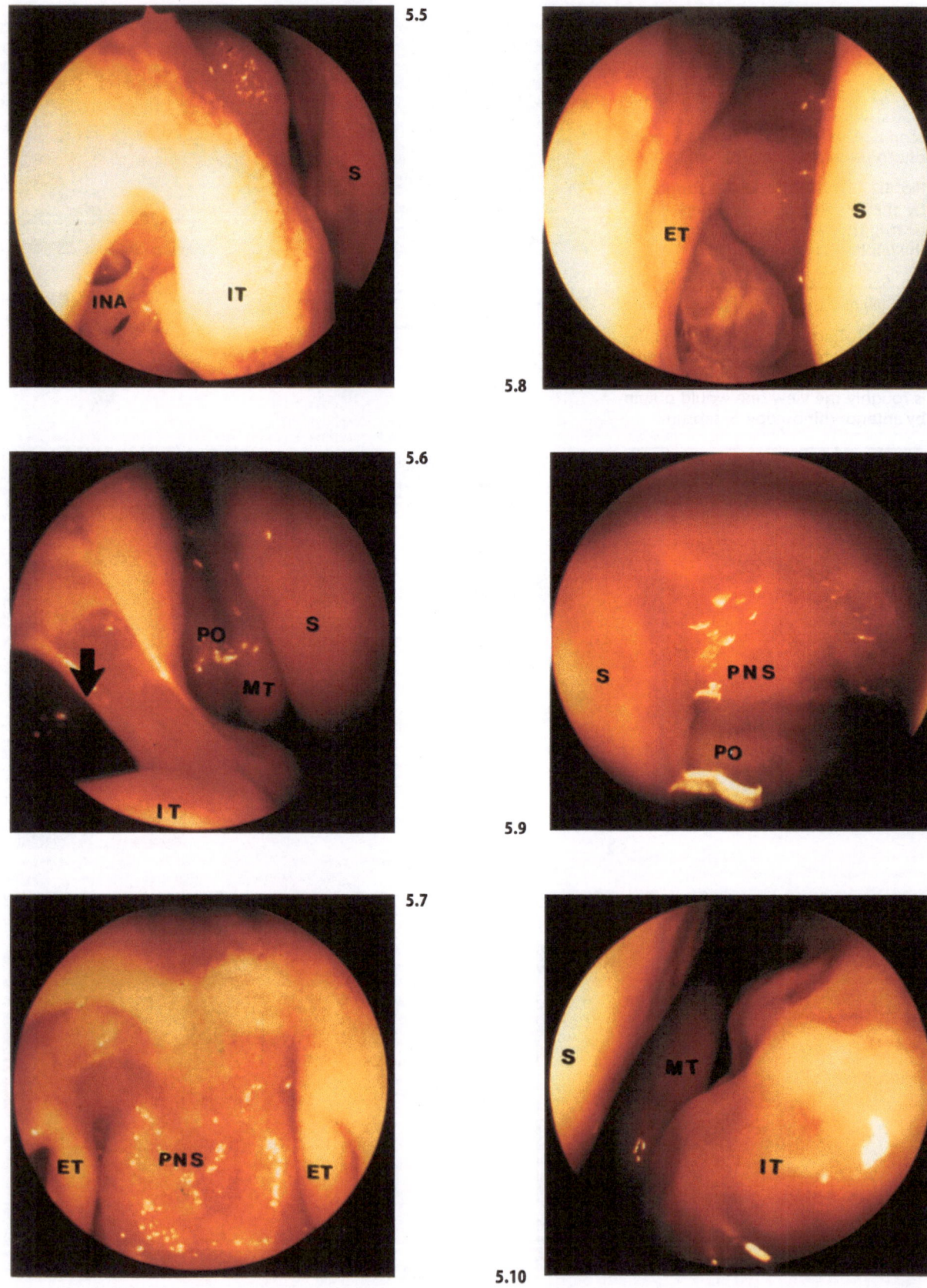

Fig. 5.5. The endoscope is guided into the inferior meatus to look for signs of previous surgery (INA, inferior nasal antrostomy). In this case, the antrostomy was quite stenosed, and the patient symptomatic.

Fig. 5.6. In this case, although the inferior-nasal antrostomy (arrow) was patent, there were polypoid (PO) changes not only inside the sinus but in the middle meatus. Once again, the patient was symptomatic. IT, inferior turbinate; MT, middle turbinate; S, septum.

Fig. 5.7. The first pass ends at the nasopharynx (PNS, post-nasal space). The eustachian tube openings (ET) are inspected. A 0° endoscope accesses the ipsilateral opening only, wheras a 30° endoscope may be rotated to visualise the contralateral side.

Fig. 5.8. Here the right first pass shows a small amount of viscous mucus emerging through the eustachian tube (ET) orifice. S, septum.

Fig. 5.9. An interesting finding. Examination of the left nasopharynx reveals an antro-choanal polyp (PO) protruding "around the bend" from the opposite side. S, septum, PNS, post-nasal space.

Fig. 5.10. The second pass begins with examination of the lateral wall of the nose. The endoscope is guided between the inferior turbinate (IT) and the septum (S) towards the middle turbinate (MT). Note the polypoidal inferior turbinate in this case.

Fig. 5.11. Very often (10%–40% of cases), an accessory ostium (AO) is seen in the anterior fontanelle. In fact, an ostium that is readily seen on the lateral wall (LW) is always an accessory one. MT, middle turbinate.

Fig. 5.12. The accessory ostium (AOS) in this case shows pus (P) tracking down from the maxillary sinus. Also note a large polyp (PO) on the floor of the nose. MT, middle turbinate; S, septum.

Fig. 5.13. The arrow demonstrates an early antro-choanal polyp protruding through the left accessory ostium. S, septum; MT, middle turbinate; AOS, accessory ostium.

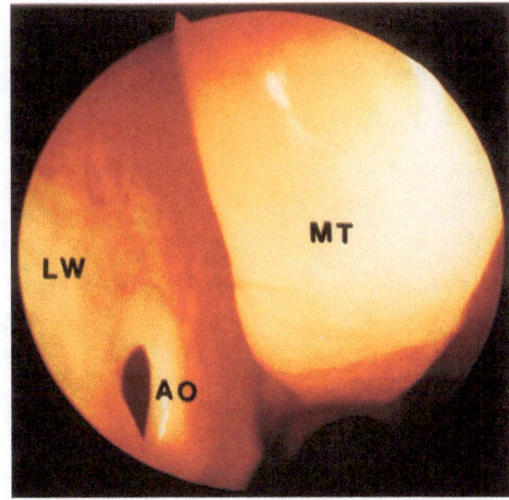

5.11

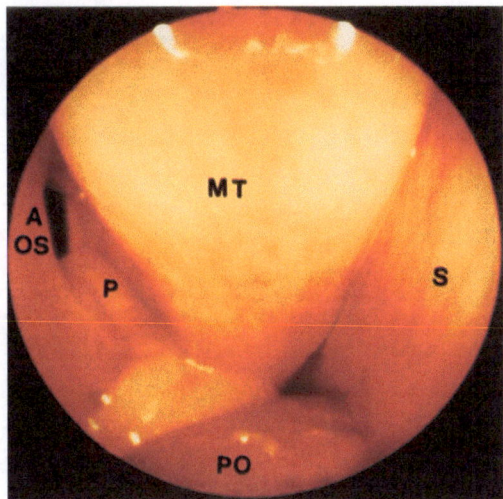

5.12

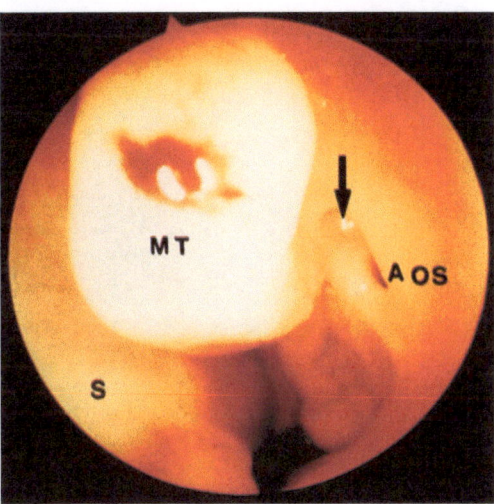

5.13

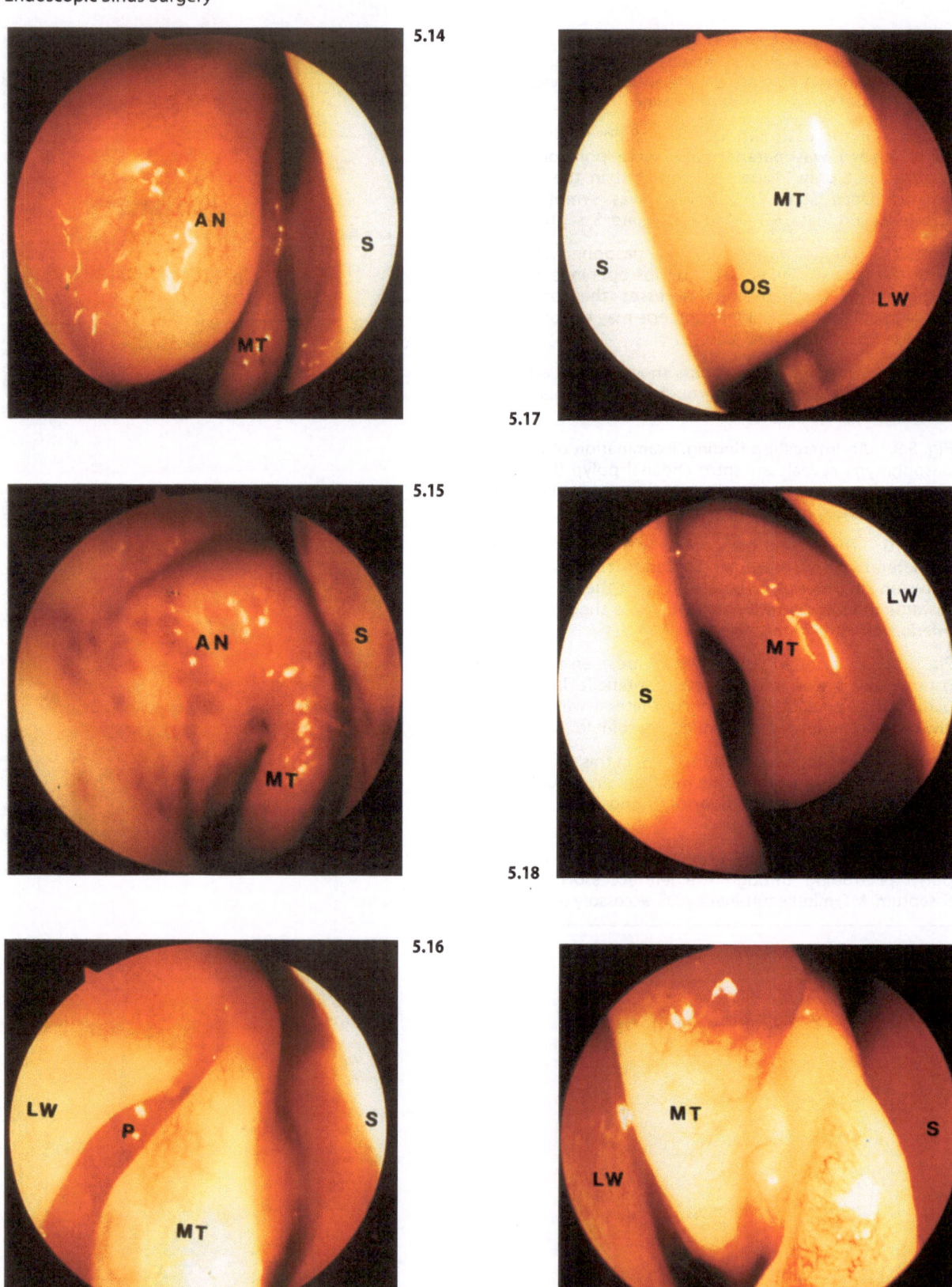

Fig. 5.14. Quite often, a bulge on the lateral wall at the attachment of the middle turbinate signifies agger nasi cells (AN). These are the most anterior ethmoid cells, often blocking the frontal recess. MT, middle turbinate, S, septum.

Fig. 5.15. Another view of the agger nasi cells (AN), chronic inflammation often causes a mottled appearance. MT, middle turbinate; S, septum.

Fig. 5.16. Endoscopic examination of the middle meatus often demonstrates minimal changes that could be causing the patient's symptoms. Here the meatus contains multiple, small polyps (P), not visible by anterior rhinoscopy. LW, lateral wall; MT, middle turbinate; S, septum.

Fig. 5.17. Deformities of the middle turbinate (MT) include pneumatisation (concha bullosa); sometimes an ostium (OS) is seen. If infected, discharge may be noticed too. S, septum; LW, lateral wall.

Fig. 5.18. The normal middle turbinate is convex medially, thus bowing away from the lateral wall (LW). Sometimes, however, this curvature is reversed, leading to a "paradoxicity" of the middle turbinate (MT). This impinges on the ostio-meatal complex. S, septum.

Fig. 5.19. At times the turbinate (MT) is bifid, and may contain air cells in one or both limbs. LW, lateral wall; S, septum.

Fig. 5.20. The middle turbinate may be bilobed (MT), giving rise to a false appearance of polyps at its anterior end, especially on anterior rhinoscopy. S, septum; LW, lateral wall.

Fig. 5.21. Endoscopy does not merely look at the lateral wall (LW); the convolutions of the septum must also be studied. Here the septum (S) shows a smooth deviation encroaching on a paradoxical middle turbinate (MT). This leads to crowding of the ostio-meatal complex.

Fig. 5.22. A sharp septal spur(s) juts out towards the middle meatus, thus causing stenosis of the ostio-meatal complex. Furthermore, apposition of mucosal surfaces causes muco-ciliary stasis often leading to oedema and polyps. MT, middle turbinate; LW, lateral wall.

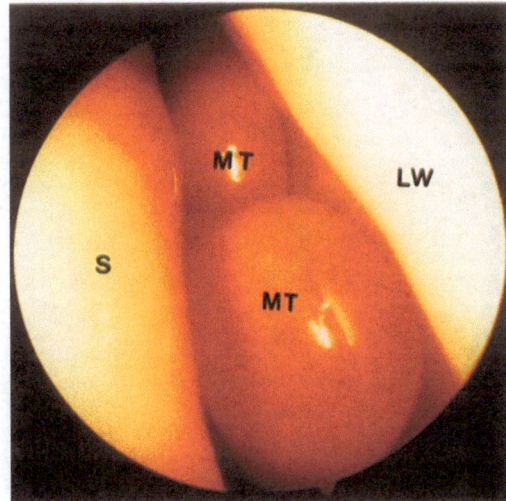

5.20

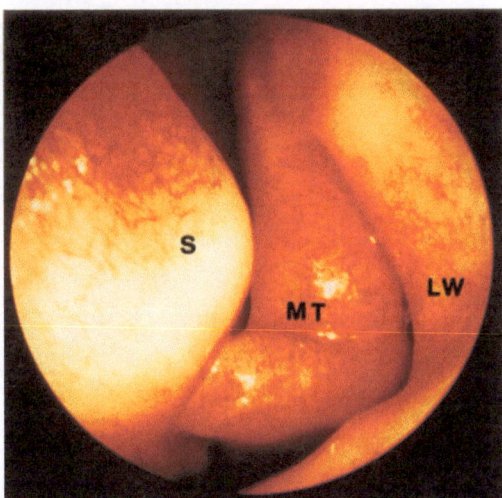

5.21

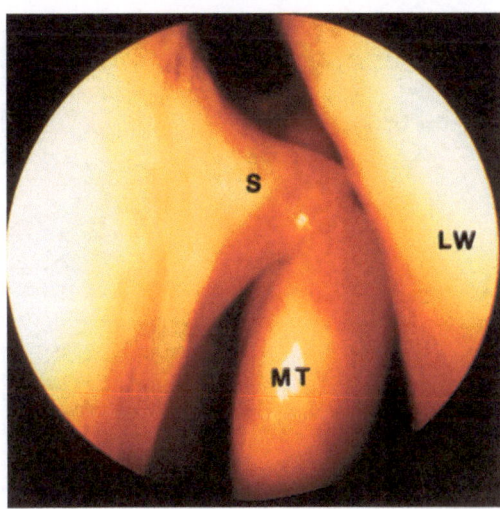

5.22

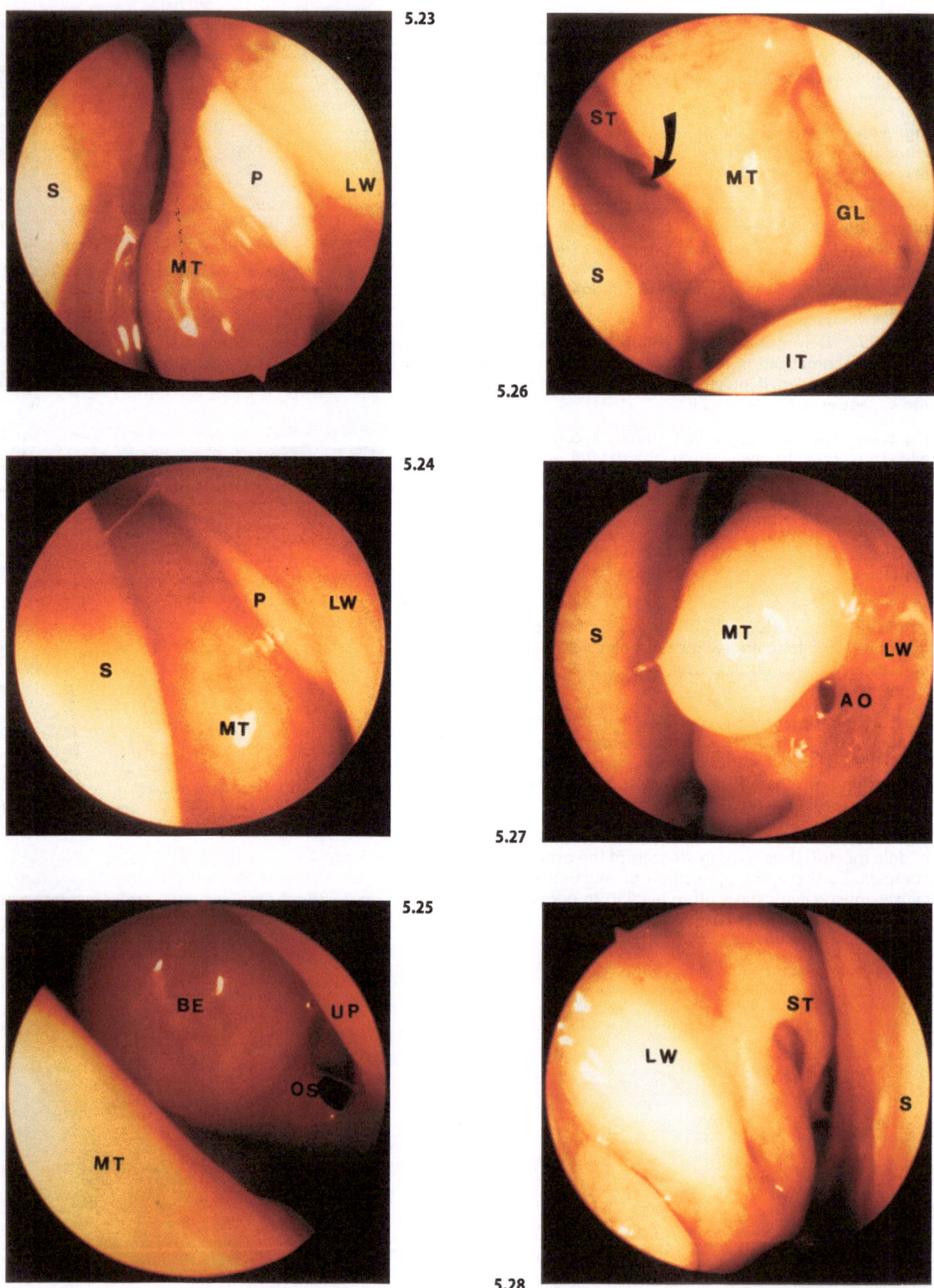

Fig. 5.23. The endoscope is now rotated into the middle meatus. Pus (P) may be seen tracking down the anterior meatal cleft, suggesting anterior sinus disease. S, septum; MT, middle turbinate; LW, lateral wall.

Fig. 5.24. Pus (P) emerging from the frontal recess is diagnostic of frontal sinusitis. S, septum; MT, middle turbinate; LW, lateral wall.

Fig. 5.25. As the endoscope enters the middle meatus, the accessory ostium (OS) comes into view. It is bounded anteriorly by the uncinate process (UP) and posteriorly by the bulla ethmoidales (BE). MT, middle turbinate.

Fig. 5.26. The posterior limit of the second pass is the ground lamella (GL) moving laterally across from the middle turbinate to the lamina papyracea. In addition, the superior turbinate (ST) and sphenoidal ostium (arrow) may be seen. S, septum; MT, middle turbinate; IT, inferior turbinate.

Fig. 5.27. Rarely, the middle turbinate (MT) may show a knobbing of its anterior end (rudimentary turbinate). Again, an accessory ostium (AO) is seen. S, septum; LW, lateral wall.

Fig. 5.28. Very rarely, the entire lateral wall (LW) may be grossly deformed, with no proper anatomical landmarks; this, of course, would make surgery hazardous. A CT is mandatory. ST, superior turbinate; S, septum.

Fig. 5.29. For a complete examination of the posterior group of sinuses, the endoscope is directed first backwards up to the posterior end of the inferior turbinate (IT), and then upwards. This brings the superior turbinate (ST) into view, along with the spheno-ethmoidal recess. PNS, post-nasal space; S, septum.

Fig. 5.30. Directing the 30° endoscope straight upwards will bring the sphenoidal recess into view (arrow). ET, eustachian tube; ST, superior turbinate; PNS, post-nasal space; S, septum.

Fig. 5.31. The third pass focuses on the superior turbinate (ST), its meatus (SM), and the spheno-ethmoidal recess. S, septum; LW, latera wall.

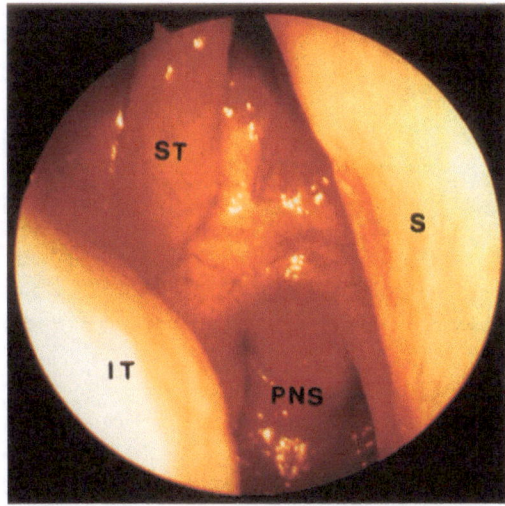
5.29

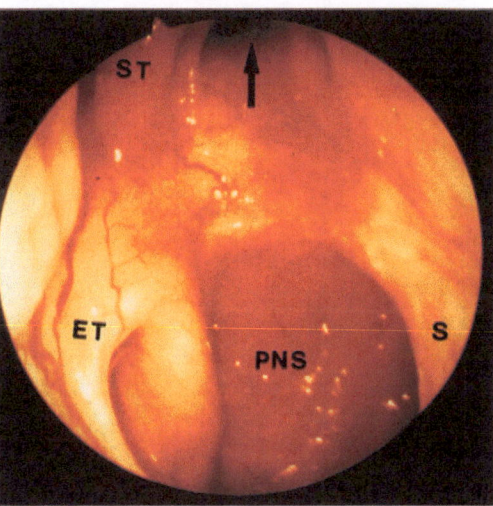
5.30

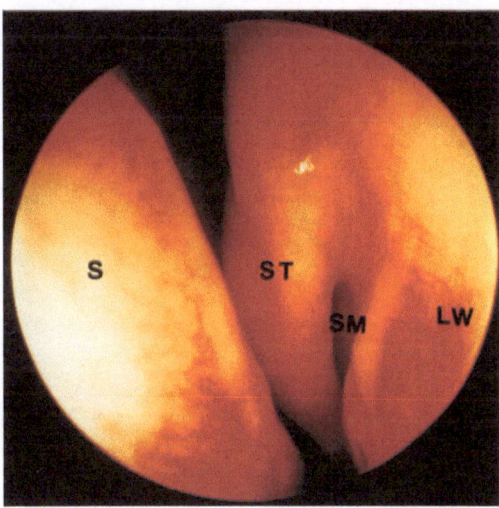
5.31

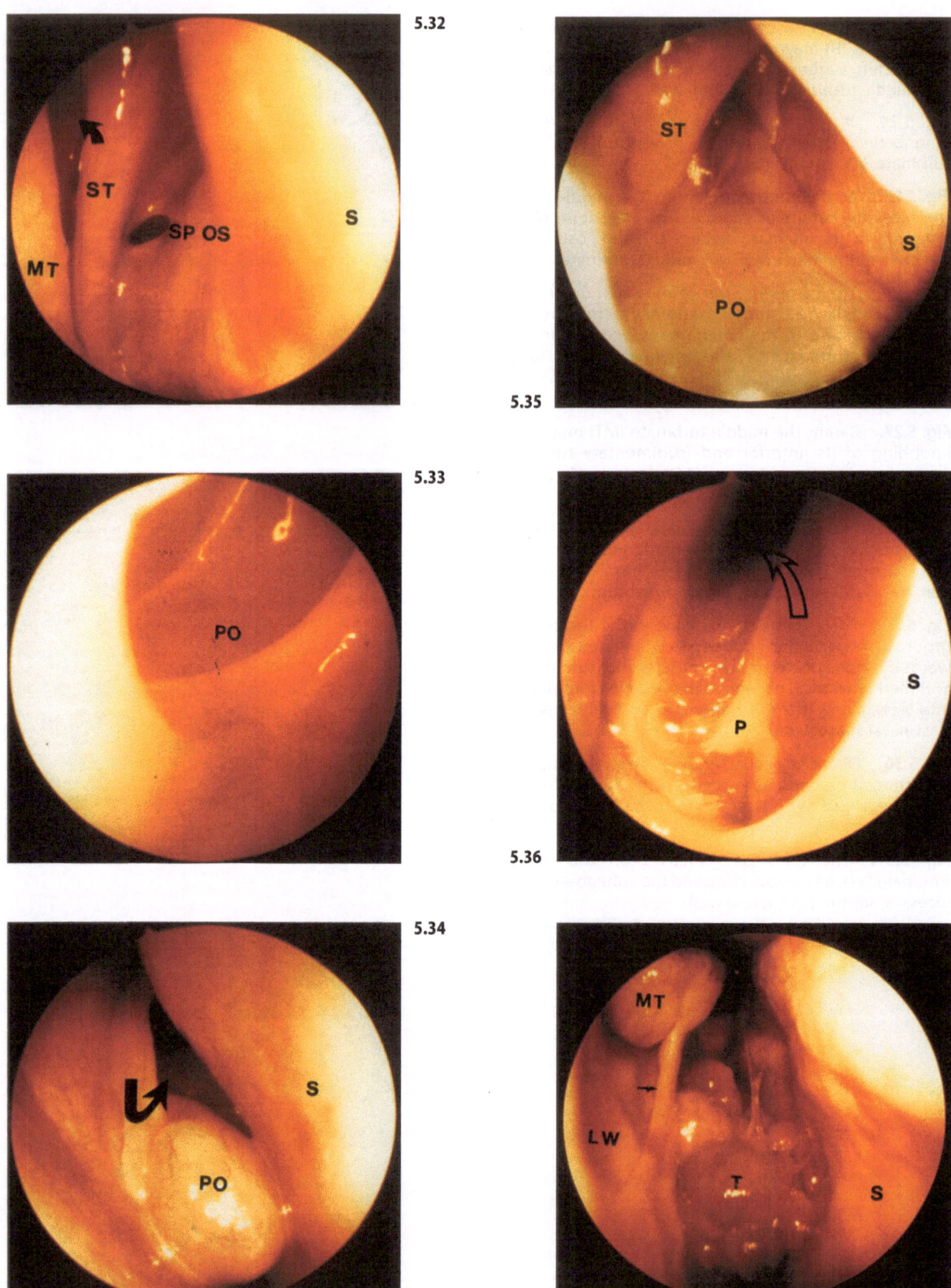

5.32

5.33

5.34

5.35

5.36

5.37

Fig. 5.32.   Further examination shows the sphenoidal ostium (SP OS), the superior turbinate (ST) and its meatus (arrow). MT, middle turbinate; S, septum.

Fig. 5.33.   Sometimes the sphenoidal ostium may be entered as in this view, showing an early polyp (PO). These patients often present as diagnostic enigmas until a throrough endoscopy reveals the true nature of the disease.

Fig. 5.34.   Similarly, examination of the superior meatus (arrow) may also reveal a polyp (PO). This indicates a posterior group disease. S, septum.

Fig. 5.35.   Pathology in the spheno-ethmoidal recess included polyps (PO), as seen emerging from the ostium. ST, superior turbinate; S, septum.

Fig. 5.36.   Further to Fig. 5.35, pus (P) may be seen tracking down from the sphenoidal ostium (arrow). S, septum.

Fig. 5.37.   Endoscopy may also be used to assess nasal tumours such as this inverted papilloma (T), which has recurred after excision several years ago. The arrow points to an adhesion due to previous surgery. LW, lateral wall; MT, middle turbinate; S, septum.

Fig. 5.38.   This patient complained of nasal obstruction and crusting. Examination showed granulations (GR) on the floor of the nose, inferior surface of inferior turbinate (IT) and septum (S) a biopsy led to a diagnosis of sarcoidosis.

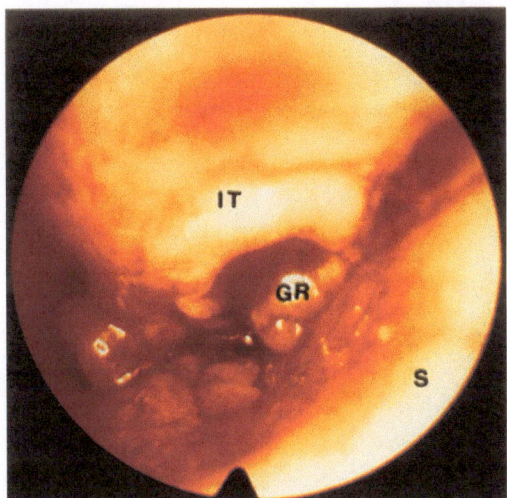

5.38

Chapter 6

Sinus Imaging

Introduction

One of the major developments in recent years has been sinus imaging with computed tomography (CT). It is now possible to study the intricate anatomy of paranasal sinuses and, more importantly, their relation to the surrounding vital structures such as skull base, lamina papyracea, internal carotid artery and optic nerve. It delineates key areas such as infundibulum and ostiomeatal complex. CT scanning is now mandatory in the pre-operative evaluation of sinus disease before undertaking functional endoscopic sinus surgery (FESS). The advent of CT scanning has significantly enhanced the scope of endoscopic sinus surgery by offering the surgeon more accurate information regarding sinus status than is possible with plain radiography.

Generally chronic sinus disease is evidenced by mucosal changes such as thickening, formation of polyps and presence of fluid levels in the sinuses.

Plain Radiography of the Paranasal Sinuses

Although CT scanning remains the investigation of choice for sinus disease, cost and availability often call for an almost reluctant reliance (on the part of the endoscopic surgeon) on plain films. Quite simply, bone throws a "shadow", while air is black, and any gradation between the two implies fluid or mucosal thickening. Thus it is a loss of translucency that characterises inflammation of the paranasal spaces. Assessment of the patient in the vertical position lets gravity enhance the information procured, as fluid levels (± menisci) are then reliably detected. Sinus views

> **CT Scan of the sinuses is mandatory in the following situations**
>
> - Children and adolescents
> - All revision paranasal sinus surgery
> - Gross nasal polyposis
> - Extensive posterior ethmoid and/or sphenoid disease as evaluated on nasal endoscopy
> - Distorted anatomy as seen on nasal endoscopy
> - Mucoceles, tumors, etc.

call for special fixation facilities of the skull to allow for standardisation of the patient/beam axis. Any deviation throws one set of sinuses away from the midline, causing a "white-out" and thus obscuring findings.

The routine views obtained are

- occipito-mental (Water's); this view demonstrates some important structures:
    - Sinuses (maxillary, postero-lateral wall, antero-lateral wall, frontal, ethmoid labyrinth
    - nasal septum
    - infraorbital foramen
    - zygoma
    - orbit

If a fluid level is suspected, it may be confirmed by tilting the head by 20–40° to the side.

- occipito-frontal (Caldwell's), this film shows
    - sinuses (frontal, maxillary, [inferior segment] ethmoid labyrinth
- lateral view, this demonstrates
    - sinuses—sphenoid, frontal, maxillary, [posterior segment]
    - floor of the anterior cranial fossa

□   orbit

□   sella turcica

■ oblique view, taken mainly for the posterior ethmoid cells and the optic foramina. The floor of the anterior cranial fossa is also seen clearly. The frontal sinuses are seen too.

The CT Scan

CT scanning of paranasal sinuses has proved the most dependable of pre-operative assessments of chronic sinus disease. By using wide and narrow window settings the bony details and soft tissue respectively can be shown precisely. Both coronal and axial scans are useful though coronal scans provide more useful information for the endoscopic surgeon.

Coronal scans have three distinct advantages over an axial scan:

1. The coronal scan illustrates progessively deeper structures encountered by the surgeon during the operation as he advances in an anterior to posterior direction, i.e. uncinate process, bulla ethmoidales, ground lamina, posterior ethmoids and sphenoid. In other words coronal scans synchronises with the steps of the operation.

2. It illucidates important relationships of the above structures to the lamina papyracea, and skull base.

3. The integrity of lamina papyracea is better appreciated in coronal scans.

It is our firm conviction that although CT is useful to elicit information about muco-periostial status, its true value lies in its ability to reflect accurately the surgical landscape of the core areas the surgeon is interested in. Both normal and variant anatomy (sinuses, ostia and intercommunicating air channels) guides one towards the cause of the patient's pathology. In our view, the scan serves as a "*road map*" for the surgeon as he negotiates the potentially hazardous clefts of the paranasal sinus unit.

We feel the primary advantage of the CT scan is the anatomical information it affords, and hence we read our films starting at the key area of the infundibular block, then moving outwards to include the para-infundibular block; finally noting the relationships of the anterior skull base and orbit to the sinuses (dehiscences of the internal carotid artery occur in a significant number of cases).

CT Scanning Technique

A coronal section CT scan is obtained in the following manner. The patient is placed prone on the scanner bed with the head hyperextended. The scanning plane is oriented so that the plane of sectioning is perpendicular to the infra-orbital meatal line. Scans are taken 3 mm apart (complete coronal section CT scan) and cover the region from the frontal sinuses to the sphenoid sinus. Bone windows (window width 4000), which are the same as those used for temporal bone imaging, are selected routinely for viewing. The selection of bone windows reduces the distortion resulting from metallic objects in comparison with soft tissue windows. It might be anticipated that a coronal section CT scan with soft tissue windows (window width 300) would be necessary in order to view soft tissue pathology; however, soft tissue/bony relationships are better demonstrated in a coronal sections with bone windows.

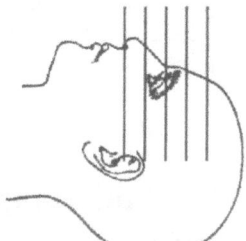

Fig. 6.1. Hyperextended head position for coronal CT scan of the sinuses.

CT Parameters

These films are used to obtain the following perspectives of the patients condition:

■ the overall extent of pneumatisation of the paranasal sinus unit, and the extent of the disease, as reflected by haziness

■ the *infundibular block*, consisting of the uncinate process, bulla ethmoidalis, the Haller cells and the middle meatus

■ the *para-infundibular block*, consisting of the middle turbinate, agger nasi cells and the lamina papyracea

■ the fovea ethmoidalis, or the floor of the anterior cranial fossa

■ the optic nerve, and its relation to the posterior ethmoid cells

■ the internal carotid artery in relation to the sphenoid sinus

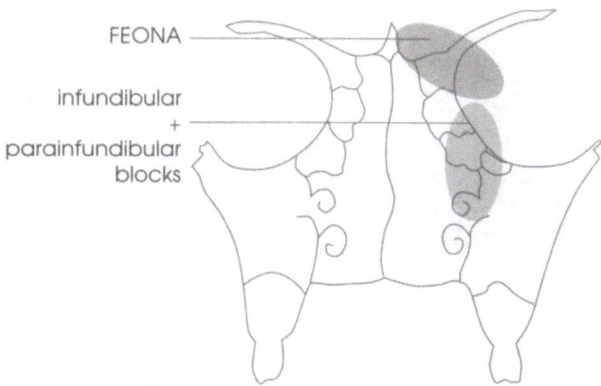

Fig. 6.2. FEONA, fovea ethmoidalis, optic nerve and internal carotid artery.

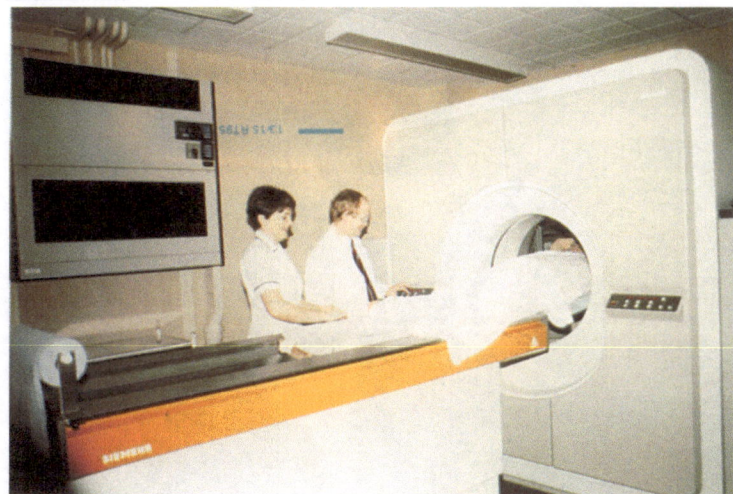

Fig. 6.3. View of a SIEMENS Somatom CR machine used for CT sinus imaging.

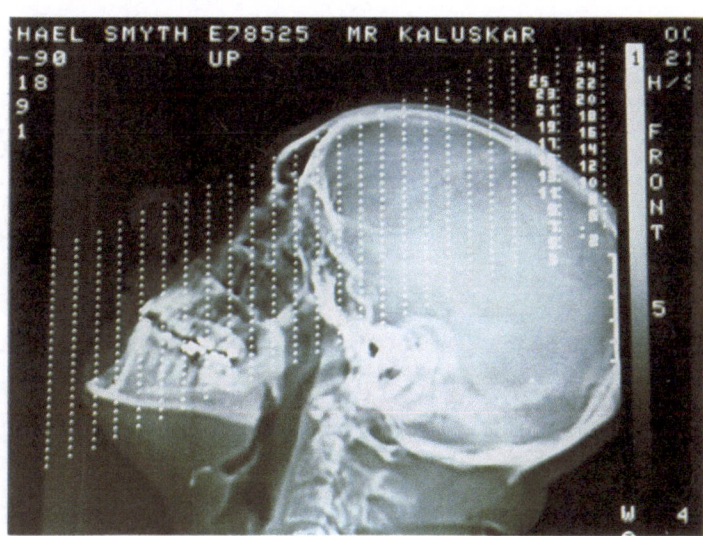

Fig. 6.4. Bone windows (3 mm) at 4-mm intervals are taken progressively from anterior to posterior for coronal CT scanning.

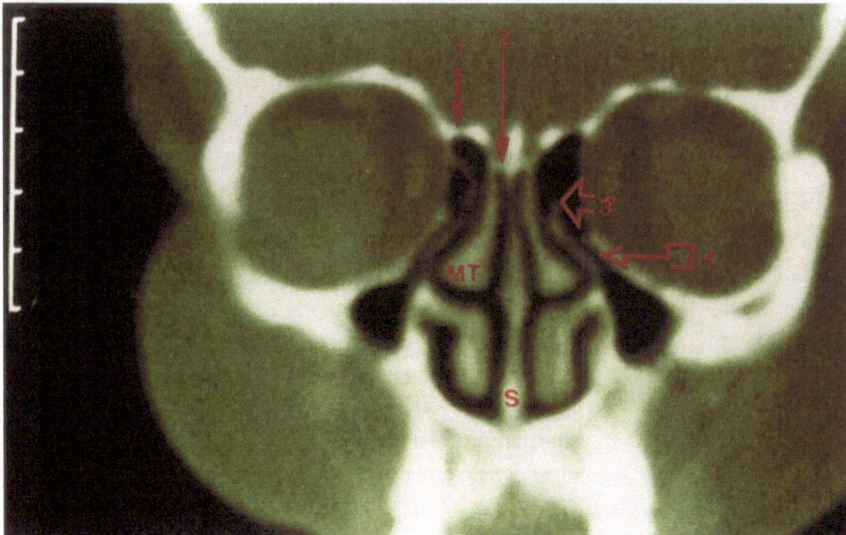

Fig. 6.5. Coronal sections reflect the surgeon's approach from anterior to posterior. More importantly, they reveal the key areas of the ostiomeatal complex as seen above (infundibular/para-infundibular blocks/FEONA). 1, the sloping roof (fovea) of the ethmoids; 2, level of cribriform plate; 3, upper limit of uncinate process; 4, infundibulum; S, septum; MT, middle turbinate.

Fig. 6.6. In a more anterior section, the fronto-nasal recess (4) could be identified easily. Other structures include: 1, sloping roof of the ethmoids; 2, cribriform plate, which descends considerably into the nasal cavity; 3, superior attachment of the middle turbinate; CG, crista galli; S, septum.

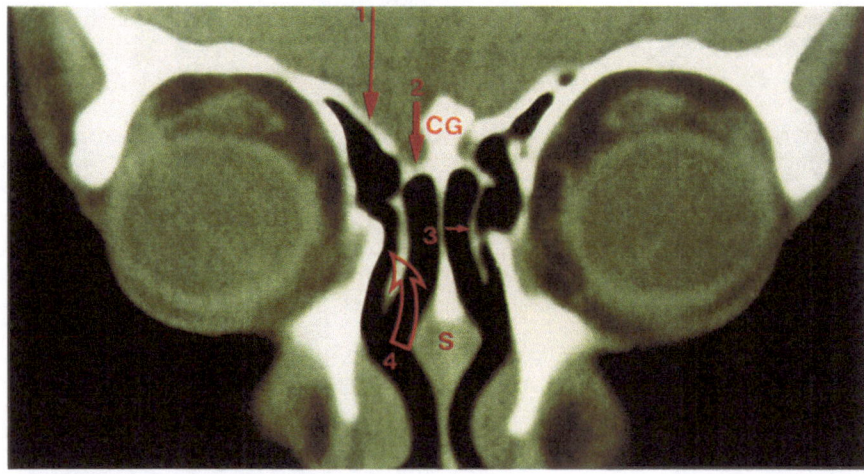

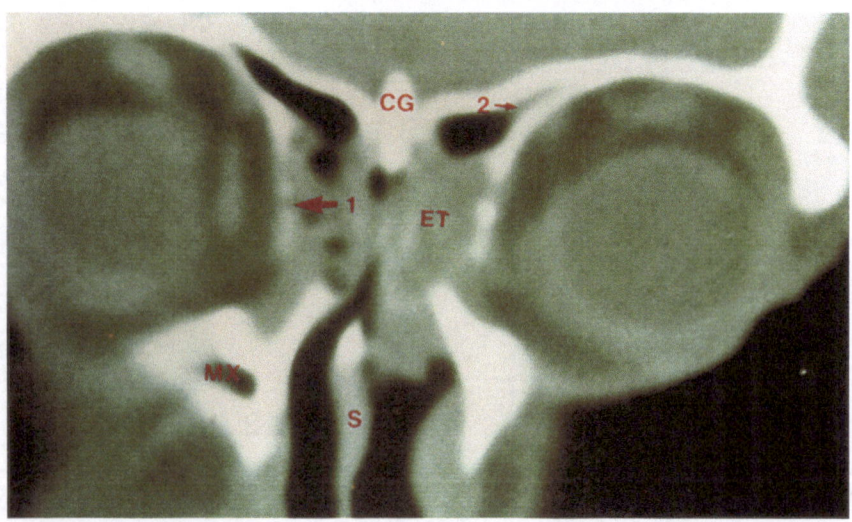

Fig. 6.7. Coronal cut through the anterior ethmoids (ET), showing extensive disease on both sides. 1, probable erosion of the lamina papyracea due to longstanding disease; 2, note disease in supra-orbital ethmoid cells; MX, maxillary sinus.

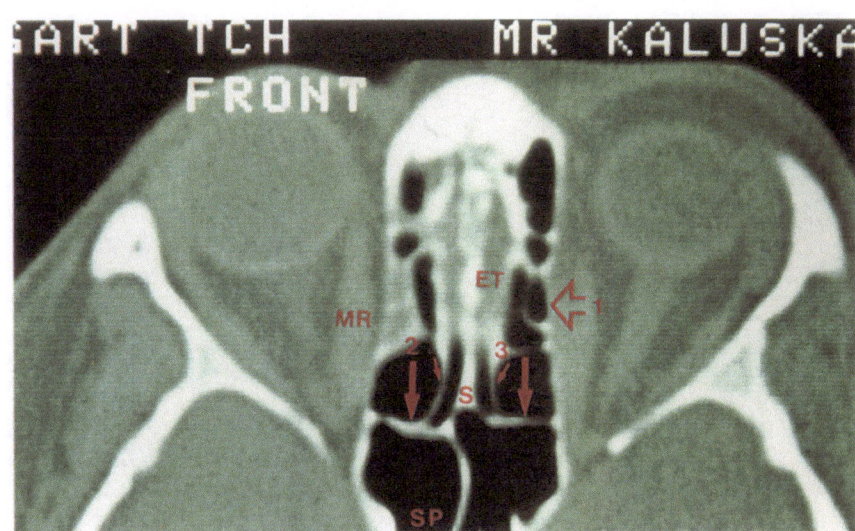

Fig. 6.8. An axial CT shows disease in the anterior and middle ethmoids. Although the relation of the orbit to the ethmoids is well seen, the important areas of the ostio-meatal complex are not seen adequately. 1, lamina papyracea separating the medial rectus (MR) from the ethmoids (ET); 2, lamellae separating the ethmoids from the sphenoids (SP) on either side; 3, upper attachments of the middle turbinate.

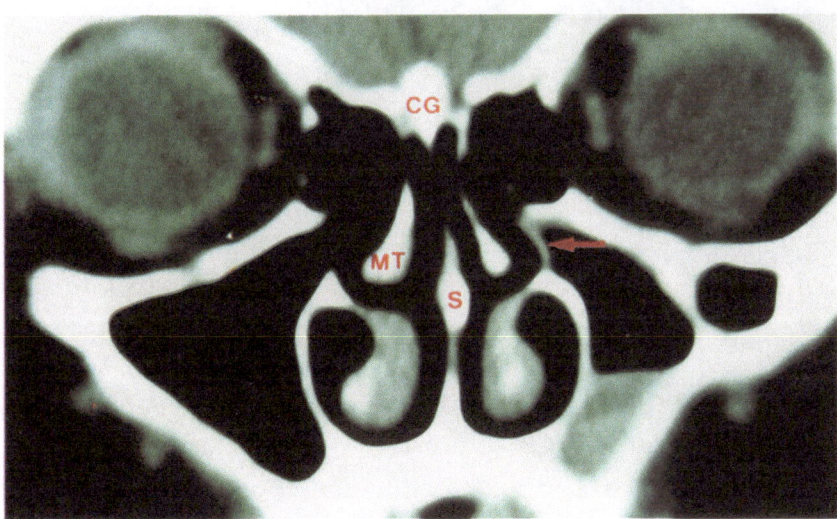

Fig. 6.9. Infundibular pathologies such as a laterally rotated uncinate process (arrow) cause stenosis of the ostio-meatal complex resulting in gross disease of the maxillary sinus. MT, middle turbinate; CG, crista galli; S, septum.

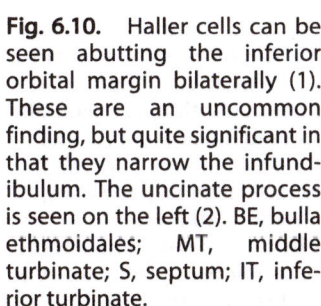

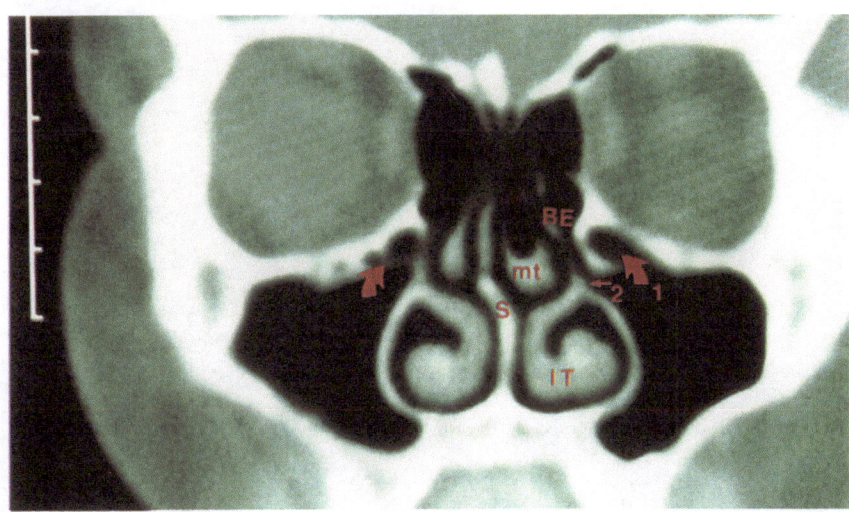

Fig. 6.10. Haller cells can be seen abutting the inferior orbital margin bilaterally (1). These are an uncommon finding, but quite significant in that they narrow the infundibulum. The uncinate process is seen on the left (2). BE, bulla ethmoidales; MT, middle turbinate; S, septum; IT, inferior turbinate.

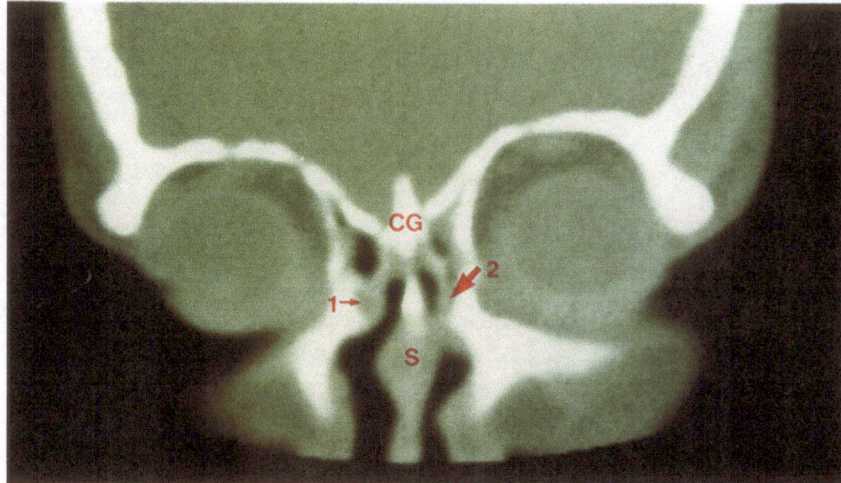

Fig. 6.11. Anterior coronal cut showing haziness in the right anterior ethmoids (1), and blockage of the fronto-nasal recess on the left (2). CG, crista galli; S, septum.

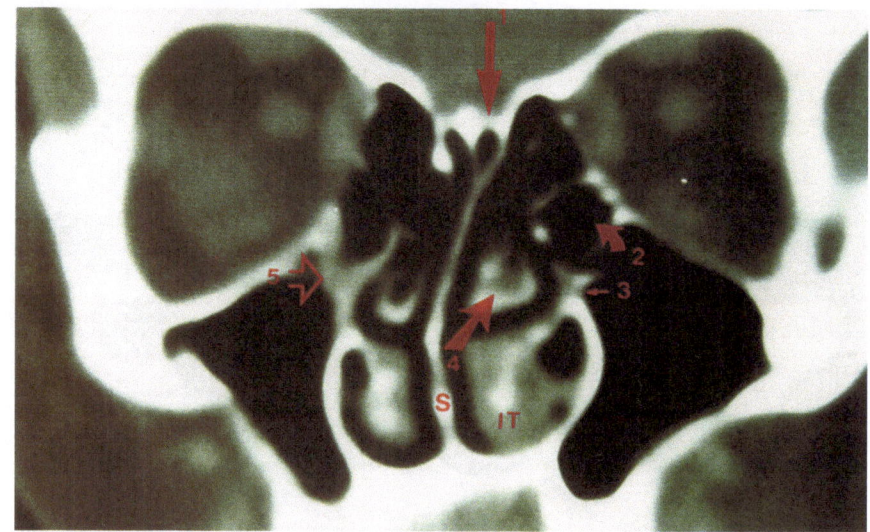

Fig. 6.12. CT scan showing several features: 1, cribriform plate; 2, large bulla ethmoidalis; 3, uncinate process; 4, haziness in a conchous left middle turbinate; 5, blocked infundibulum on the right. S, septum; IT, inferior turbinate.

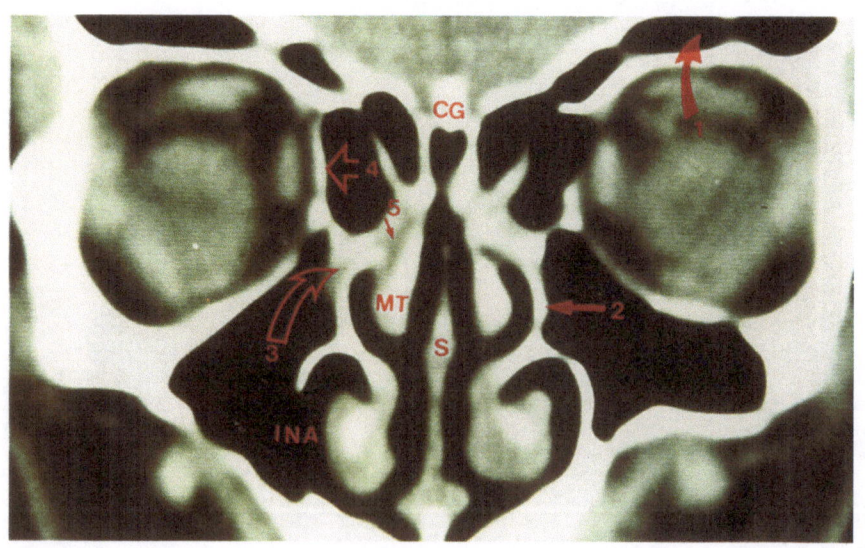

Fig. 6.13. Anterior cut showing several important features: 1, extensive supra-orbital pneumatisation; 2, laterally rotated uncinate process; 3, blocked, narrow infundibulum; 4, lamina papyracea; 5, anterior ethmoidal disease; INA, inferior nasal antrostomy. MT, middle turbinate, CG, crista galli; S, septum.

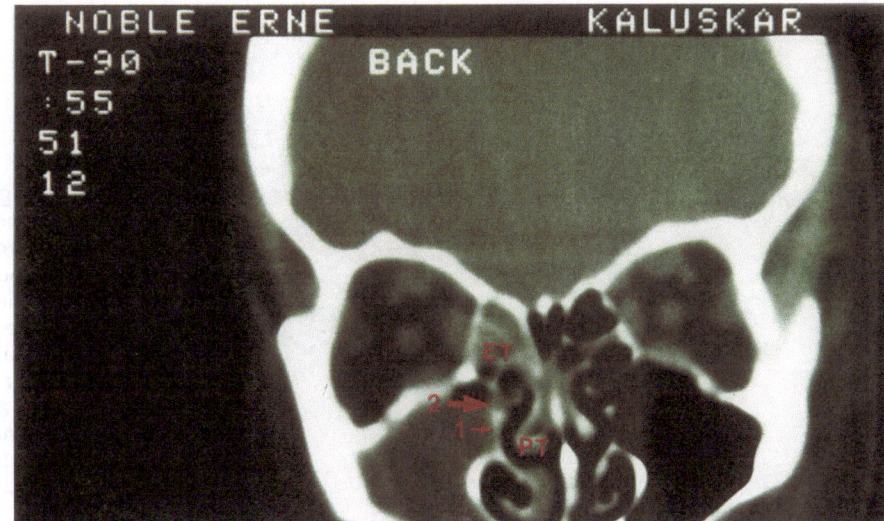

Fig. 6.14. Unusual, unilateral pan-sinusitis showing a paradoxical turbinate (PT) in association with ethmoidal (ET) and maxillary disease. 1, uncinate process; 2, blocked infundibulum.

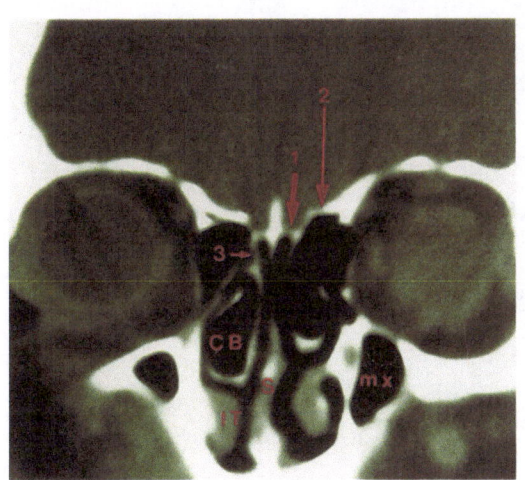

a

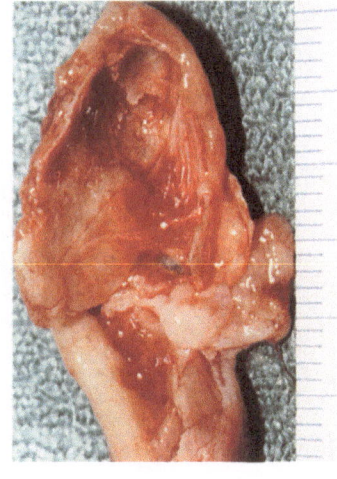

b

Fig. 6.15. **a** Right concha bullosa (CB), note its lateral wall encroaching on the OMC. 1, cribriform plate; 2, fovea ethmoidales; 3, superior attachment of the middle turbinate. IT, inferior turbinate; S, septum; MX, maxillary sinus. **b** Post-operative specimen of excised concha bullosa.

Fig. 6.16. Another common abnormality is the paradoxical turbinate, seen here bilaterally (1); 2, roof of the ethmoids; 3, cribriform plate. ET, ethmoids; S, septum.

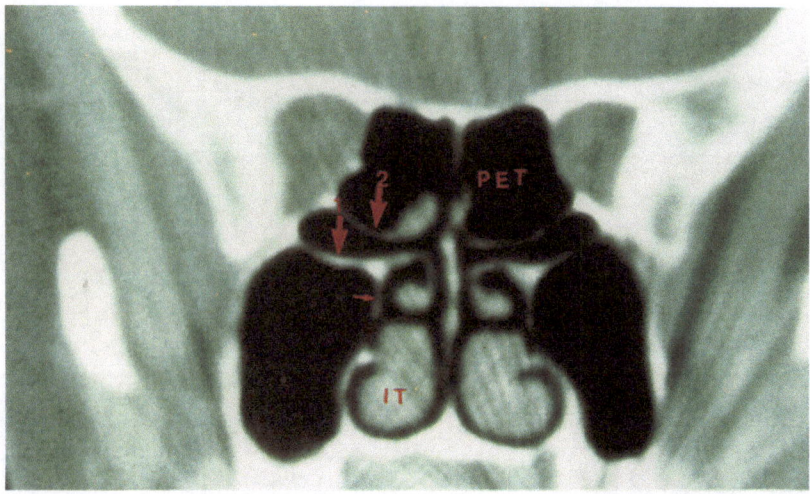

Fig. 6.17. Further posterior cuts show up a series of sequential ground lamellae, separating ethmoid cell planes. In this section, the main ground lamella (1) can be seen extending from the middie turbinate to the medial wall of the orbit. Just behind this is another lamella (2). Small arrow, uncinate process; PET, posterior ethmoids; IT, inferior turbinate.

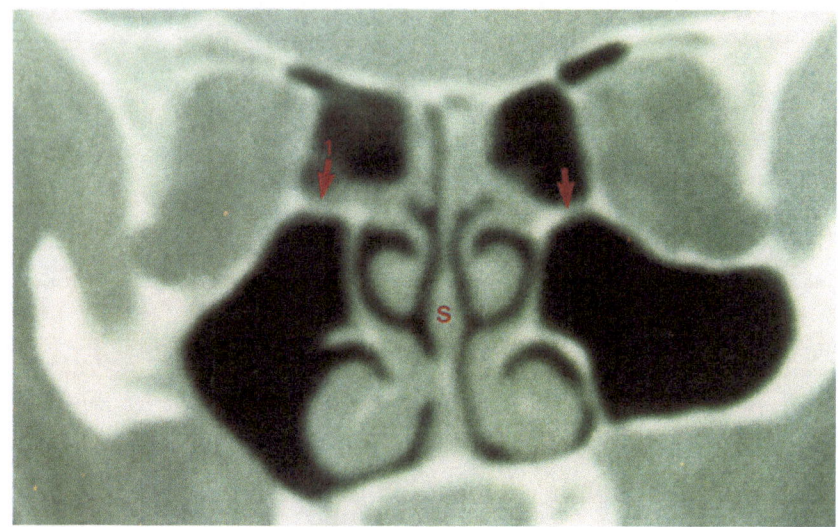

Fig. 6.18. The main ground lamella (1) is seen, note posterior cell disease. S, septum.

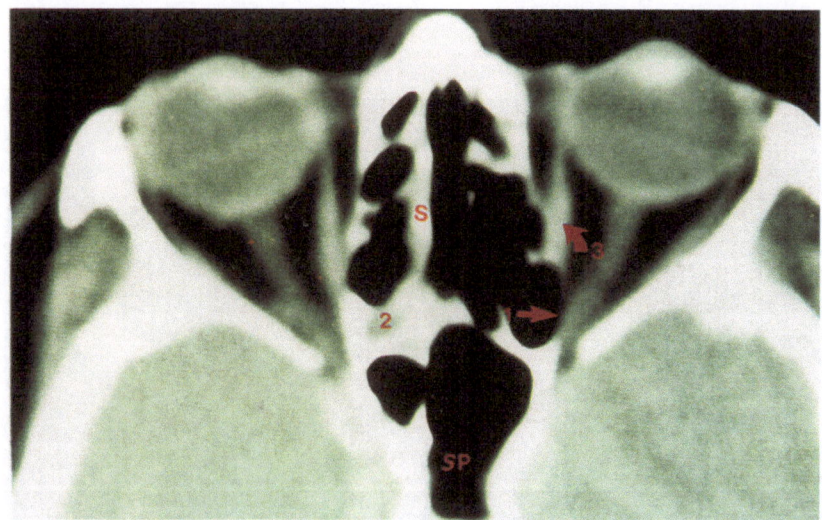

Fig. 6.19. Axial scan showing Onodi cell (lateral extension of the posterior ethmoidal cell) (1), thus exposing the optic nerve directly to the operative field. Note the posterior ethmoid disease on the opposite side (2). 3, medial rectus; SP, sphenoid sinus; S, septum.

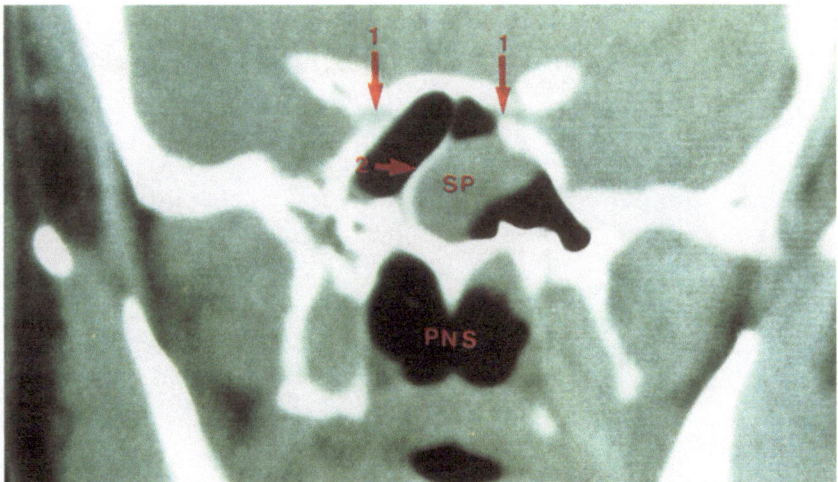

Fig. 6.20. Sphenoid cuts showing haziness in the left sphenoid sinus, along with dehiscences of both internal carotid arteries into the sphenoidal lumen (1). This is a not uncommon finding and, therefore, sphenoidal disease should be treated with extreme care. 2, inter-sphenoid septum. SP, sphenoid sinus; PNS, post-nasal space.

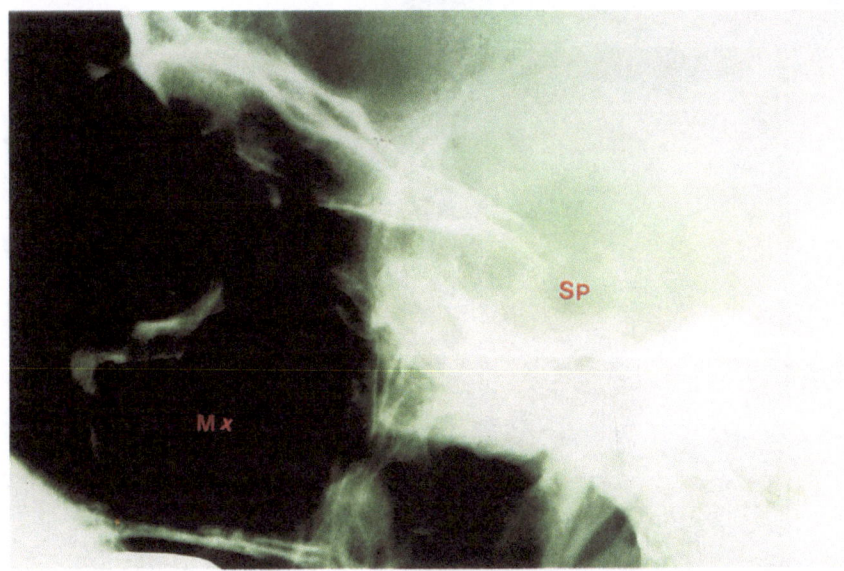

Fig. 6.21. This patient suffered from severe headaches, the only positive finding was a haziness of the sphenoidal sinus. MX, maxillary sinus; SP, sphenoid sinus.

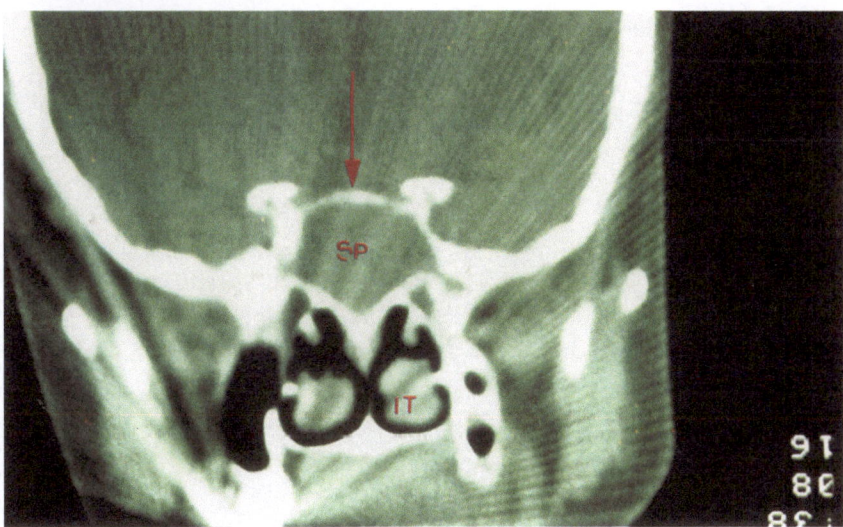

Fig. 6.22. The coronal CT scan revealed bowing of the posterior wall of the sphenoid sinus (arrow). Endoscopic removal confirmed a mucocoele. SP, sphenoid sinus; IT, inferior turbinate.

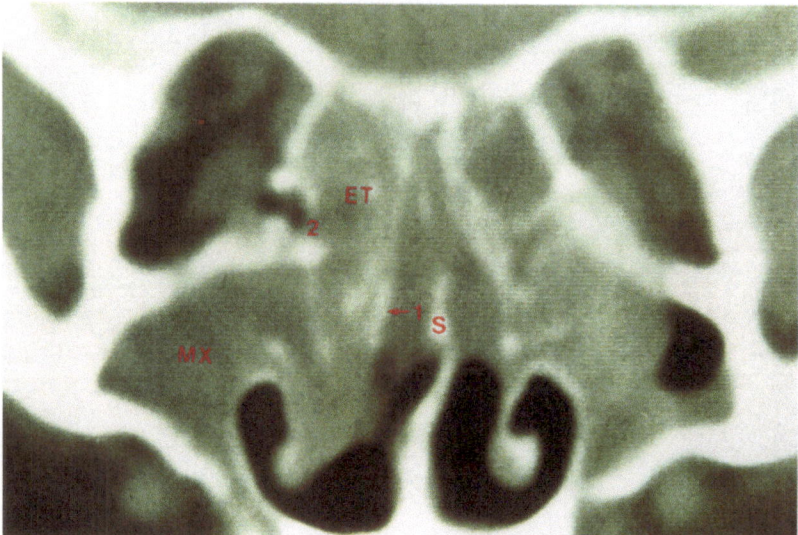

Fig. 6.23. This is a case of extensive, recurrent, bilateral pan-sinusitis. The patient underwent several polypectomies to no avail. There is complete distortion of surgical landmarks. Only remnants of the right middle turbinate could be seen (1), and there was an erosion of the lamina papyracea (2). CT results such as these should serve as warning lights, an external ethmoidectomy would be the preferred option for all except the truly experienced. MX, maxillary sinus; ET, ethmoids; S, septum.

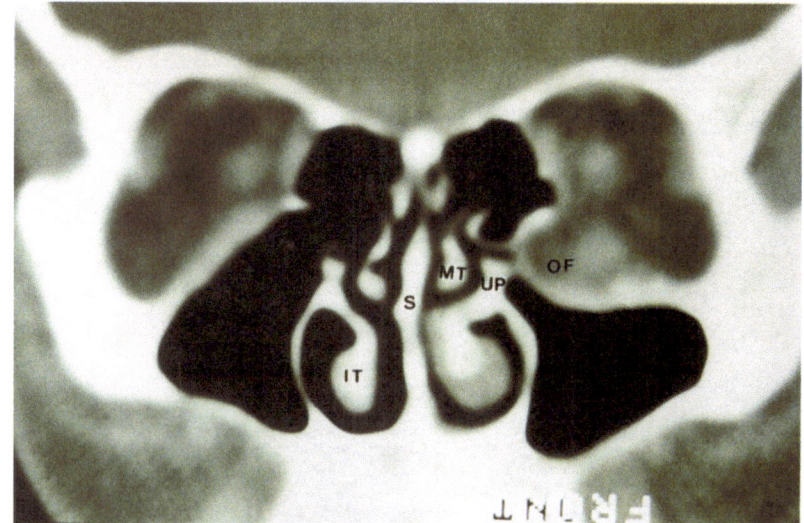

Fig. 6.24. Coronal CT scan showing inferior turbinate (IT), septum (S), middle turbinate (MT), uncinate process (UP) and orbital fat (OF) prolapsing into the infundibulum due to dehiscence of the lamina papyracea. The patient suffered from a blow-out orbital fracture.

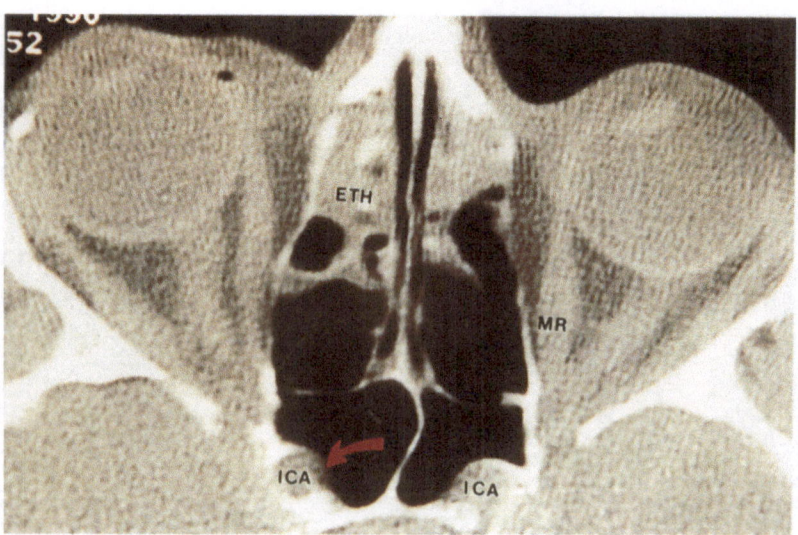

Fig. 6.25. Axial CT scan of the sinuses showing medial rectus muscle (MR), internal carotid artery (ICA) and dehiscence of the internal carotid artery in the lateral wall of the splenoid sinus (arrow). ETH, ethmoid sinuses showing mucosal disease.

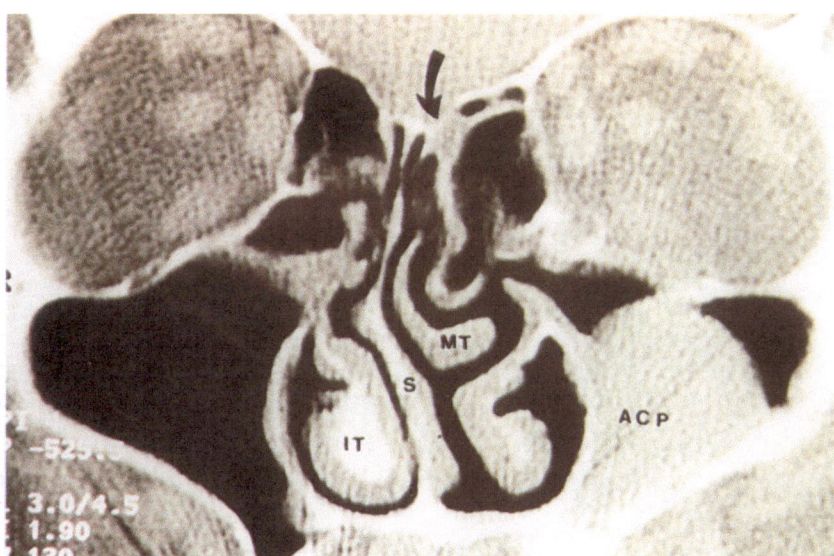

Fig. 6.26. Coronal CT scan of the sinuses. IT, inferior turbinate, S, septum; MT, middle turbinate; ACP, antrochoanal polyp. The arrow shows dehiscence of the lateral lamella of the cribiform plate.

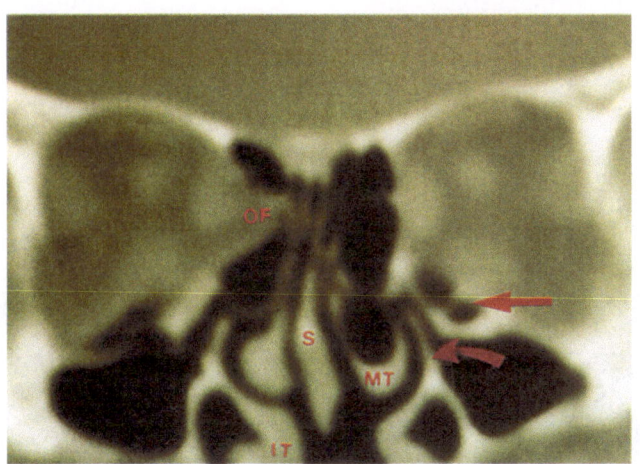

Fig. 6.27. Coronal CT scan. OF, prolapsed orbital fat in the ethmoid sinus due to dehiscence of the lamina papyracea; S, septum; MT, pneumatised middle turbinate (concha bullosa); IT, inferior turbinate; straight arrow, Haller cell; curved arrow, uncinate process.

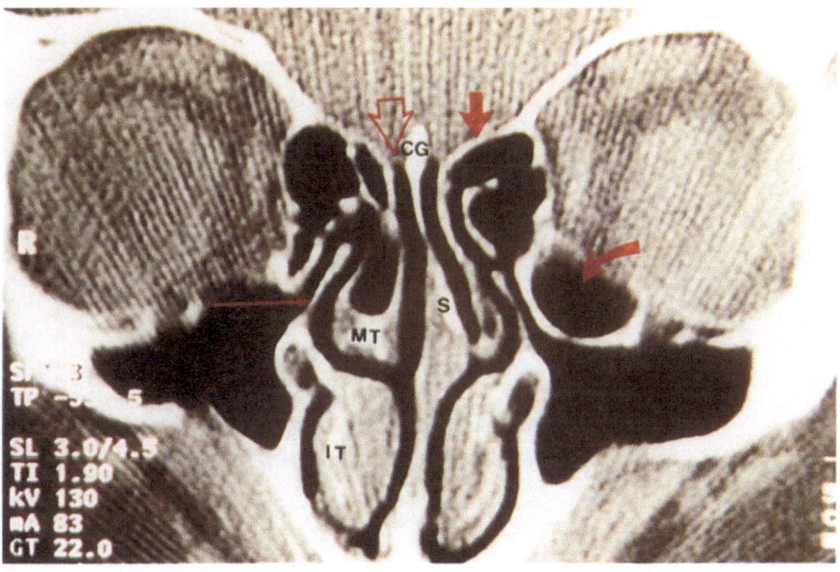

Fig. 6.28. Coronal CT scan of the sinuses. CG, crista galli; S, septum; MT, middle turbinate; IT, inferior turbinate; long arrow, uncinate process; hollow arrow, thin medial part of the fovea ethmoidales; short arrow, lateral part of the fovea ethmoidales; curved arrow, Haller cell, narrowing infundibulum.

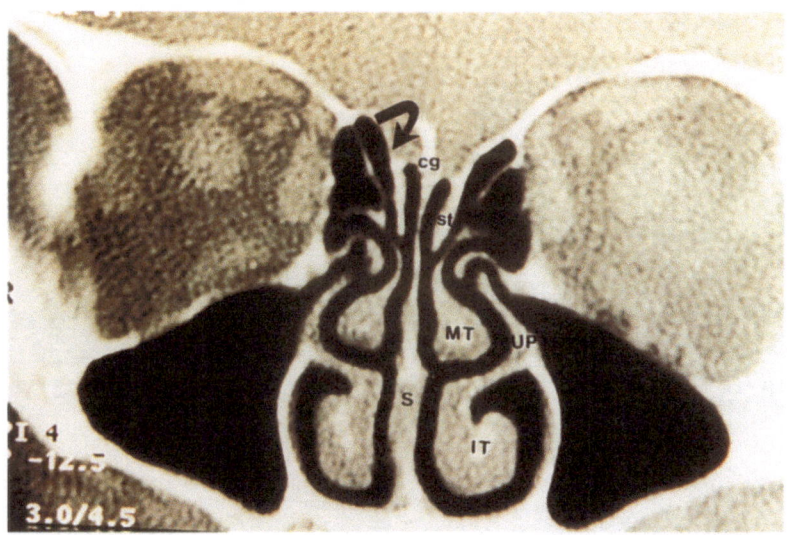

Fig. 6.29. Coronal CT scan. CG, crista galli; ST, superior turbinate; MT, middle turbinate; UP, uncinate process; IT, inferior turbinate; S, septum; arrow shows thin lateral lamella of the cribiform plate.

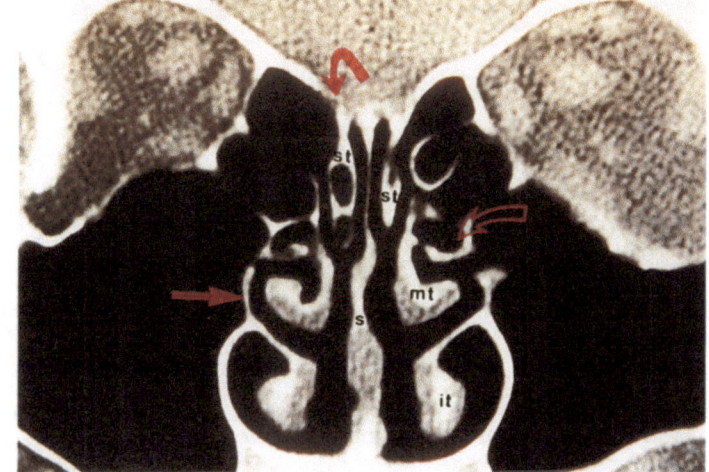

Fig. 6.30. Coronal CT scan of the sinuses. S, septum; IT, inferior turbinate; MT, middle turbinate; ST, superior turbinate (note pneumatisation); hollow arrow, bulla ethmoidales; curved arrow, dehiscent lateral lamella of the cribiform plate; straight arrow, uncinate process.

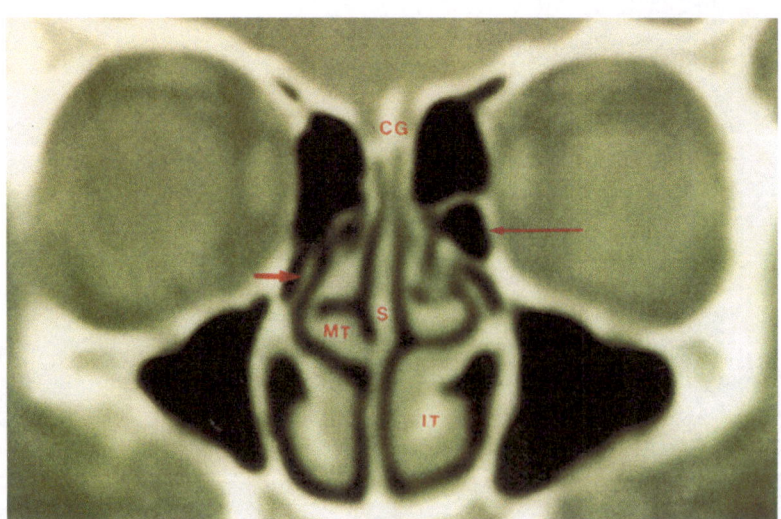

Fig. 6.31. Coronal CT scan. CG, crista galli; S, septum; MT, bifid middle turbinate, adherent to the septum; IT, inferior turbinate; short arrow, uncinate process; long arrow, bulla ethmoidales.

Why CT?

- diagnosis: confirmation or exclusion
- extent of pneumatisation
- anatomical relations with orbit/ anterior/cranial fossa
- structural abnormalities: uncinate process/concha bullosa/bulla ethmoidales/Haller cell/hypoplastic sinus, etc.
- "road map" for the surgeon

When CT?

- when the patient is not symptomatic
- treatment with antibiotics and decongestants for at least 3 weeks is recommended prior to CT

Frequent discussions regarding scans with the radiologist are recommended!

Plain films versus CT scans

On comparing the two investigations, we have found a good correlation (70%) between plain radiographs and CT scans for the maxillary sinus. The remaining 30% largely consists of patients in whom there is evidence of maxillary sinus disease on plain films, but their CT results are quite normal. This is probably due to the thickness of surrounding bone and soft tissue shadow giving an erroneous diagnosis of sinus infection on plain films. Similarly, the sphenoid sinus is clearly read on both plain films and CT scans (showing a correlation of 80% in our series); most of the remaining 20% are 'false' positive plain films.

Ethmoid sinus assessment proves more complicated. Fig. 6.32 shows the correlation between plain films and CT scans in a sample of 100 consecutive CT scan/plain film sets we analysed.

As can be seen, there is a significant risk of plain films not reflecting the true status of the sinuses in that they are under-read. Overall, 57 cases showed no correlation between the two modalities. Frontal sinus analysis produced a similarly mixed picture although the overall correlation was 67% (Fig. 6.33).

To sum up, the frontal and maxillary sinuses tend to be over-read on plain views, while the ethmoids tend to be under-read. As this is the key area of dysfunction in most cases of chronic rhinosinusitis requiring surgery, the value of plain radiographs as a pre-operative tool seems limited to gross anatomical discrepancies and acute infections with fluid levels.

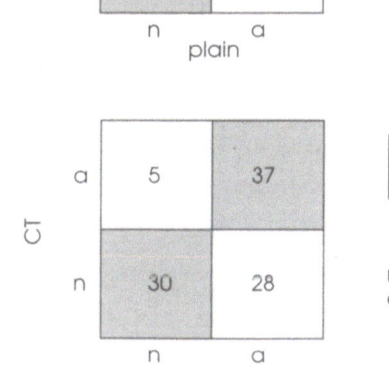

Fig. 6.32. Correlation between plain films and CT scans for ethmoid disease.

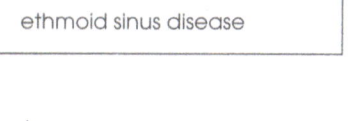

Fig. 6.33. Correlation between plain films and CT scans for frontal disease.

CT versus Operative Findings

In our experience, operative findings in the maxillary sinuses tend to correlate well with CT. For the ethmoids, however, we find that mucosal disease tends to be far more widespread than is detected on CT: It is essential, therefore, to be cautious regarding even seemingly insignificant changes in the infundibular and para-infundibular blocks.

Chapter 7

Medical Aspects of Sinusitis

Introduction

Sinusitis is an inflammation involving the mucous membrane of the paranasal sinuses. The cause is most often a respiratory virus, with secondary bacterial infection although a variety of other agents play a significant role. The clinical profile may range from a mild nasal stuffiness to severe, debilitating disease. Complications may be associated with significant morbidity and mortality.

Pathogenesis

Sinuses are lined with pseudostratified columnar ciliated epithelium, and drain through ostia into the nasal cavity. This drainage is dependent upon the functional patency of the ostium, which is more important than its anatomical size. Normal sinus clearance further depends on muco-ciliary integrity and action. Thus, any dysfunction of ostial patency, mucus production or ciliary action will increase the risk of sinusitis. Finally, hypoxia of the sinuses could further predispose to subsequent sinusitis.

The most crucial parameter in the pathogenesis of sinusitis appears to be the patency of the ostium. The normal size of the os varies for the different sinuses but may be as small as 1–2 mm (the usual diameter of an ethmoid cell ostium). The ostium may decrease further in size under certain normal circumstances such as being in the recumbent position. Other factors include

- inflammation and oedema associated with viral upper respiratory tract infections or allergic rhinitis
- local pathology such as:
  - nasal polyps
  - septal spurs/deviations
  - tumours
  - barotrauma
  - foreign bodies
  - dental abscesses
- focal pathology:
  - primary ciliary dyskinesias
  - Young's syndrome
  - cystic fibrosis
  - Kartagener's syndrome

In patients with these conditions, both the quality and the quantity of mucus production are deranged. For example, the mucus produced by cystic fibrosis patients is very viscid, and this probably accounts for the high incidence of sinusitis.

Muco-ciliary transport may be affected by ciliary dyskinesias – poor co-ordination of ciliary beat patterns may be found. Mucus is normally moved toward the ostia by the beating motion of the ciliated lining cells. Impairment of the nasal ciliary motility can be temporarily induced by viral infections, temperature changes, chemicals and certain drugs. Sinus infection causes a quantitative loss of cilia which is normally reversible, but if severe purulent rhino-sinusitis with scarring occurs this loss may be permanent, with ciliated epithelium replaced by squamous epithelium.

Immunoglobulins such as IgA, IgG and IgM are found in low concentrations in purulent secretions; thus, patients with hypogammaglobulinaemia are at risk for sinusitis.

Normal ventilation of the sinuses is important for mucosal aeration. There is a direct correlation between the ostial size and oxygen tension in the sinus. When the ostium is patent, the PO_2 is around 115 mmHg. The PO_2 falls with obstruction and may be reduced almost to zero in the setting of purulent sinusitis, with a concomitant increase in PCO_2. Anaerobic growth is encouraged by low oxygen tension. In patients with recurrent sinusitis, oxygen tension in the sinuses is reduced chronically *even when the sinus is infection-free*. Generalised causes of sinus compromise include:

- acquired immunodeficiency syndrome (AIDS), both T-cell and B-cell defects occur
- diabetes, which especially predisposes to sinus fungal infections

Bacteriology

Until recently, it was thought that the symptomatic paranasal sinus was sterile; with the advent of better aerobic and anaerobic laboratory techniques there is sufficient evidence to suggest that "normal flora" exist in the sinuses. Sinus aspiration often shows anaerobic isolates, predominantly *Bacteroides* sp. (over 50% *B. melaninogenicus*), anaerobic gram-positive cocci, and *Fusobacterium*. Predominant isolates among the aerobes are beta- and alpha-hemolytic strept ococci, *S. pneumoniae*, *Haemophilus influenzae* and *Staphylococcus aureus*.

Clinical Features of Chronic Sinusitis

The signs and symptoms of chronic sinusitis are often non-specific and difficult to differentiate from the common cold, influenza-type syndromes or allergic rhinitis. Purulent nasal discharge and facial pain or tenderness are the most common features of the disease. Additionally one might see disorders of smell, nasal congestion, cough or a history of recent upper respiratory tract infection.

The symptom profile in chronic sinusitis may be summarised as in Fig. 7.1.

Treatment

Although this book deals predominantly with functional endoscopic sinus surgery (FESS), we would like to emphasise that all patients must first be vigorously and adequately treated with medication. The principles of treatment are:

- eradicate infection (antibiotics)
- establish drainage and ventilation (systemic/local decongestants)
- treat underlying predisposing factors

Antibiotic therapy in sinusitis should, as always, be directed against the most common pathogens *Streptococcus pneumoniae*, *Haemophilus influenzae* and *Branhamella catarrhalis*. Empirical therapy is appropriate as sinus punctures are not routinely indicated except in complicated or refractory cases. Ampicillin, amoxicillin, cephalosporin group and trimethoprim/sulphamethoxazole have all been shown to be of use. The

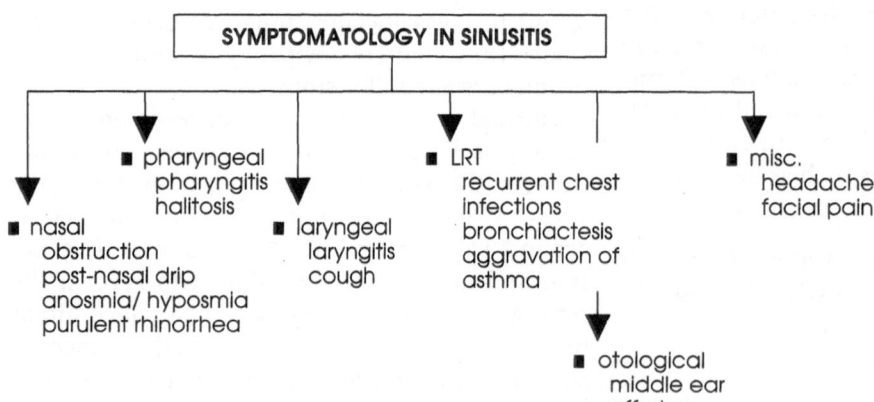

Fig. 7.1. Multiple symptoms of chronic sinusitis.

duration of the therapy should be at least 3 to 4 weeks. In addition to antibiotics, oral decongestants and steroid nasal sprays are commonly used. Inhalations help to loosen secretions. Antihistamines are of value in allergic patients. If a gram-negative result is returned by the laboratory, anaerobes and resistant gram-negative bacilli should be suspected, especially in chronic sinusitis. The cephalosporin group of drugs and metronidazole are of use in these cases. Mycotic sinusitis is a more morbid condition, often requiring surgical debridement plus systemic anti-fungals such as amphotericin B. FESS is considered in those patients who do not respond to medical management, and who have sinus disease as evinced by history of recurrent sinusitis, office endoscopy with or without CT scanning.

Acute Sinusitis: Summary

Causes

- upper respiratory tract infection
- entry of infected water during swimming/ diving
- dental extraction in the presence of root infection
- fractures involving the sinuses

Predisposing Factors

- local: obstruction of the nose, e.g. deviated septum, pathology of the ostio-meatal complex
- general: chilling, fatigue, atmospheric pollution

Clinical Features

Clinical features vary with the intensity of infection and efficacy of drainage.

- stabbing pain over the infected sinus, aggravated by bending or coughing
- muco-purulent discharge
- nasal obstruction (due to mucosal swelling)
- tenderness over the affected sinus
- oedema of the overlying soft tissue
- constitutional symptoms, e.g. pyrexia, malaise

Treatment

- systemic antibiotics (broad spectrum penicillin)
- analgesics
- restoring drainage of the affected sinus by systemic decongestants and/or irrigation. Endoscopic management of acute conditions should only be undertaken by an experienced practitioner.

Chapter 8

FESS Technique

Introduction

The two classic endoscopic approaches are those of Messerklinger (1985) and Wigand (1978). The Wigand technique calls for a back-to-front exenteration of disease from the paranasal sinuses, while the Messerklinger approach deals with the anterior group of sinuses unless there is definite evidence of posterior group disease in which case a complete fronto-ethmoido-sphenoidotomy and frontal sinusotomy could be performed. Both aim at re-establishing normal drainage channels, thereby reversing the diseased mucosa to normalcy; – the latter technique, however, is more widely practised the world over. We have based our technique on that of Messerklinger, as a vast majority of our patients present with early disease. The Wigand technique finds application in cases of massive polyposis or in revision surgery (where anatomical landmarks are distorted).

Both local and general anaesthetic are used for our patients. We prefer local anaesthesia, as there is significantly less bleeding. An awake patient is his own best guardian: any manoeuvring in the region of the orbit or the anterior cranial fossa elicits immediate pain in spite of adequate sedation and thorough topical anaesthesia! A general anaesthetic is therefore reserved for apprehensive patients, or those in whom a concomitant procedure such as septoplasty and/or rhinoplasty is required.

Local Preparation

Patients are operated on on a day-care basis, i.e. they are admitted on the morning of the operation, and leave that very evening.

The patient is positioned as shown in Fig. 8.1, and his or her clinical proforma and CT scan are made available. Sedation is achieved with Benzodiazepines derivative. The nose is prepared using serial cotton wool strip or soft universal strippacks soaked in 4% cocaine + 1:1000 adrenaline. The cavity is filled from anterior to posterior and inferior to superior. On average, preparation takes 20–30 minutes in all. Once extensive decongestion is achieved, specific blocks are targetted towards the following:

■ posterior end of middle turbinate *the spheno-palatine ganglion*

■ junction of nasal bone and upper lateral cartilage *anterior ethmoidal nerves*

■ middle meatus

The third block is an added precaution in case the spheno-palatine block is not satisfactory because of poor access to the region. Finally, the area of the uncinectomy on the lateral wall of the nose is

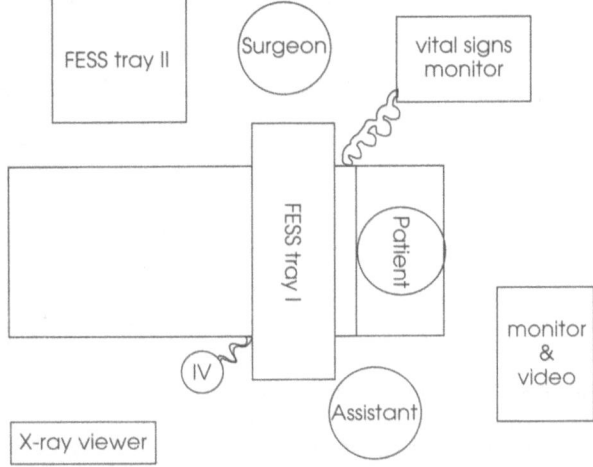

Fig. 8.1. Operating theatre set-up and layout for a patient operated on under local anaesthesia.

infiltrated with 0.5 ml of 1% lignocaine with 1:200,000 adrenaline so the anterior end of the middle turbinate is also infiltrated, especially when a concha bullosa needs to be tackled.

FESS Technique

Adequate access to the ostio-meatal complex is of vital importance to the surgeon, and hence any FESS procedure must begin only after correction of relevant septal deformities (caudal and/or high septal deviations), if any. Also, external architecture defects such as osteo-cartilaginous complex deformities should be taken care of by a functional rhinoplasty before endoscopic work commences.

The patient is placed in the 20° head-up position with the neck slightly flexed. This also brings the anterior cranial fossa into a more vertical plane. This means that when instruments are inserted posteriorly, they are less likely to be near the anterior cranial fossa. The procedure may be started using either the 0° or 30° endoscope; we prefer the former. As a first step, the middle turbinate is medialised gently, so that the middle meatus can be comfortably accessed.

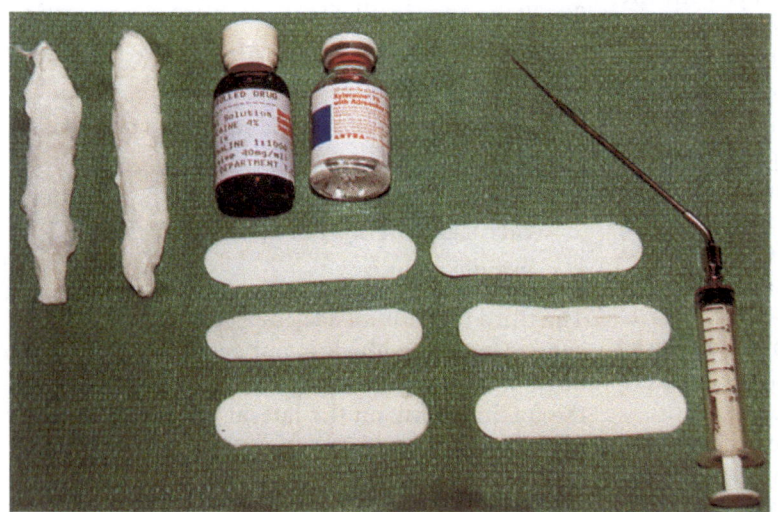

Fig. 8.2.   A strip of cotton wool soaked in 4% cocaine/ adrenaline and carefully squeezed before use. In addition, 1% lignocaine with 1 : 200 000 adrenaline is infiltrated into the operative field.

Fig. 8.3.   After initial preparation of the nose, further blocks are applied with cotton wool applicators soaked and squeezed in 4% cocaine/adrenaline to the three sites (spheno-palatine nerves, anterior ethmoidal nerve, middle meatus) on each side.

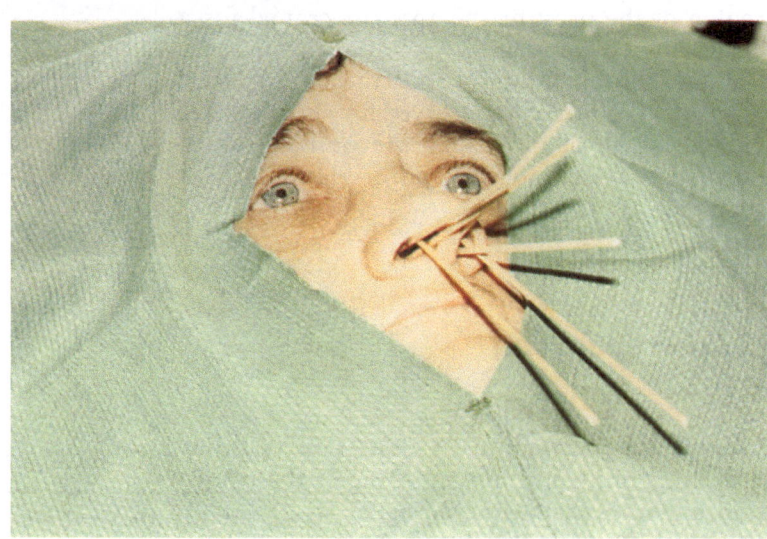

8.4

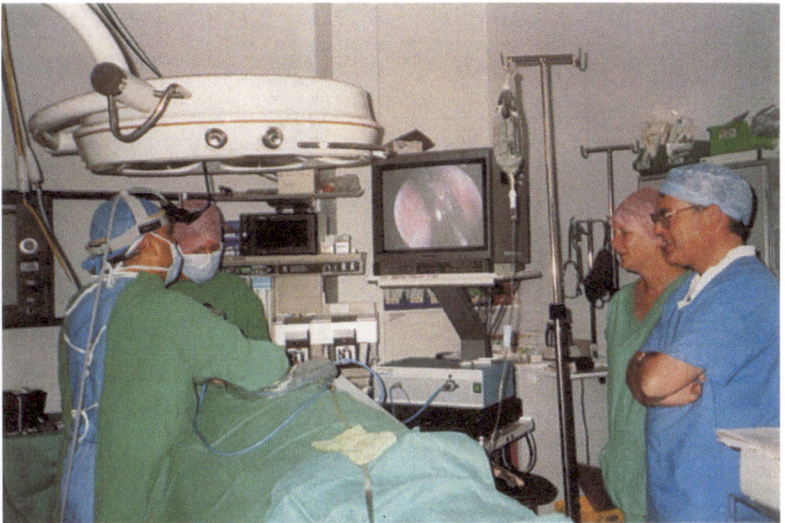

Fig. 8.4. A local FESS in progress. The patient is given an intravenous sedative, and is monitored for vital functions.

Fig. 8.5. Often a concomitant procedure such as septorhinoplasty is performed in order of: 1, septoplasty; 2, hump removal; 3, tip rotation; 4, FESS; 5, osteotomies.

Fig. 8.6. Gentle medialisation of the middle turbinate is the first step of the operation. LW, lateral wall; UP, uncinate process; MT, middle turbinate; S, septum.

Fig. 8.7. Seen here is the site of incision (arrows), between the caudal border of the uncinate process (UP) and the cephalic border of the fronto-nasal process. LW, lateral wall; MT, middle turbinate; S, septum.

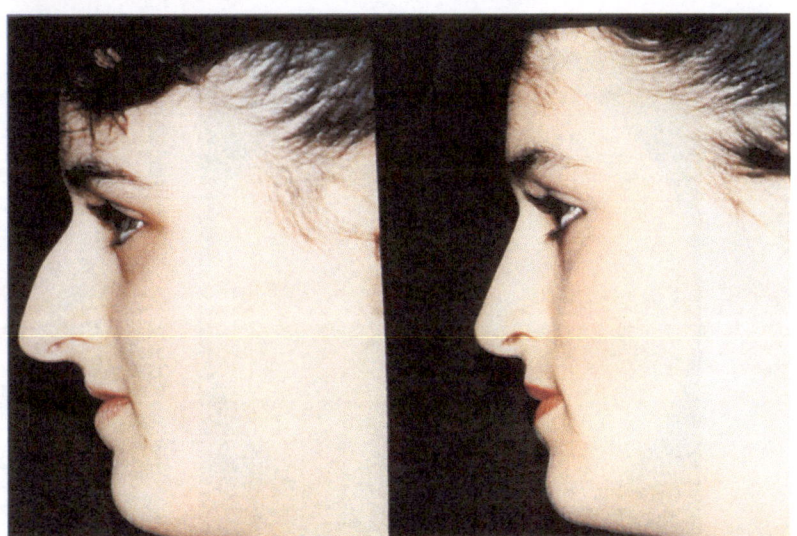

8.5

8.6

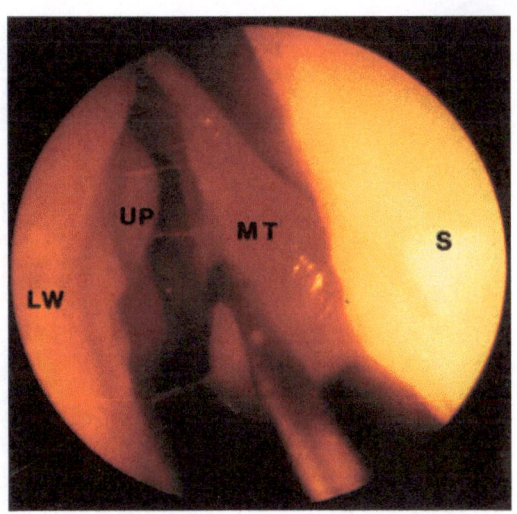

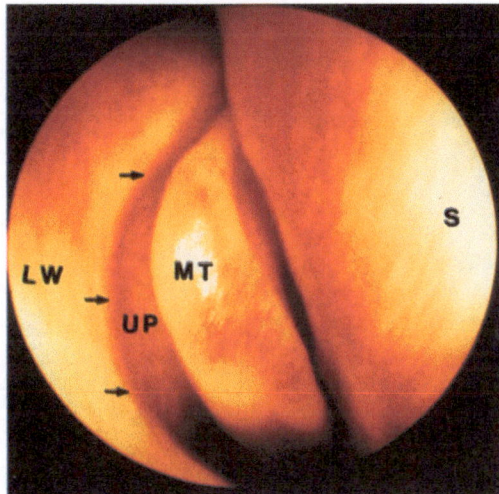

8.7

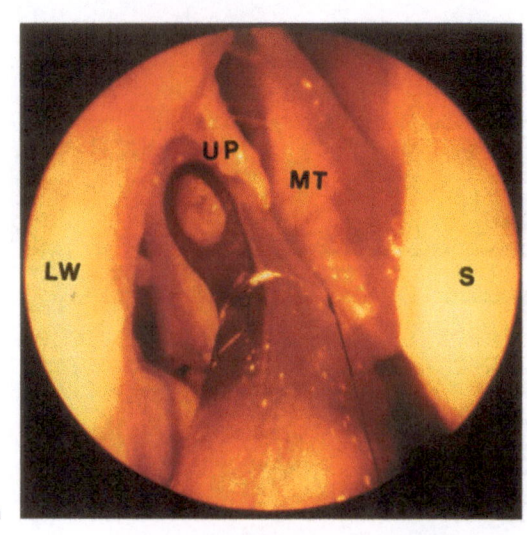

a

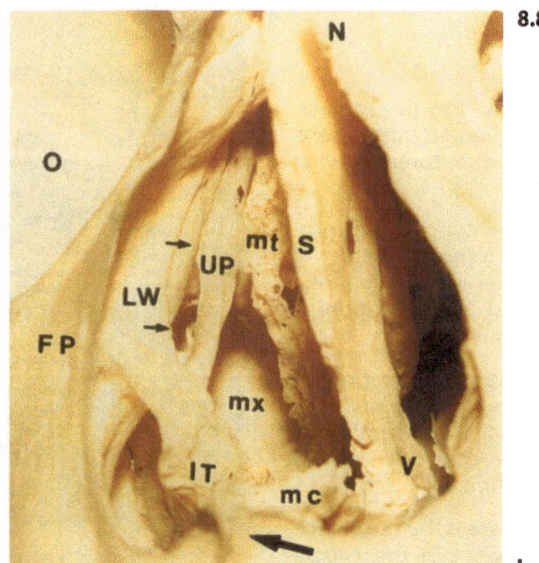

8.8

b

8.9

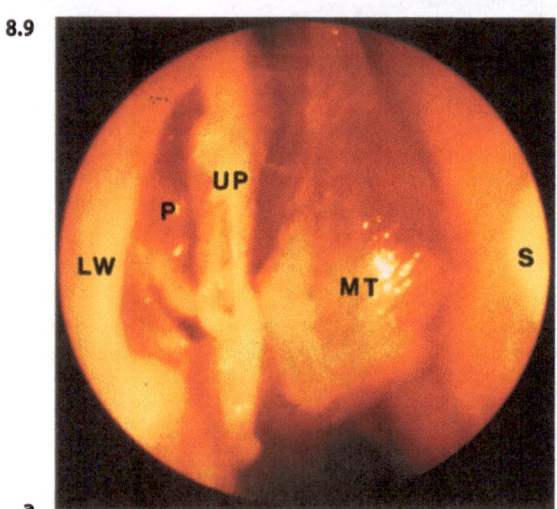

a

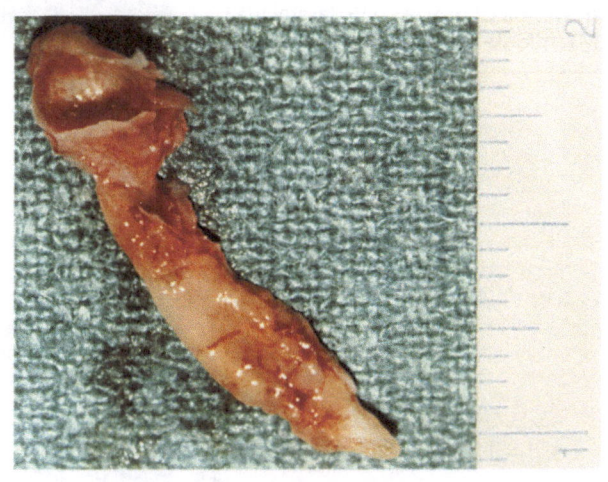

b

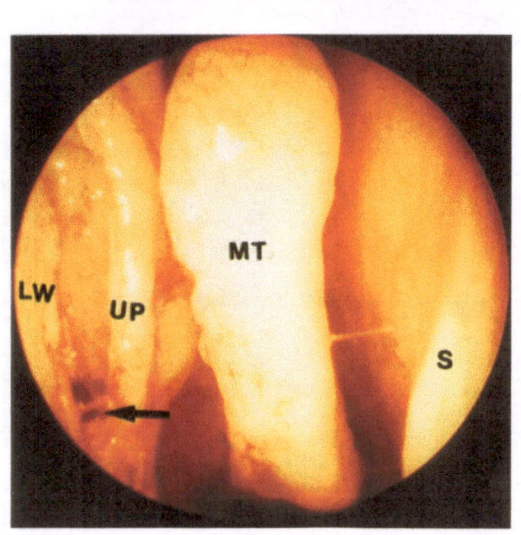

8.10

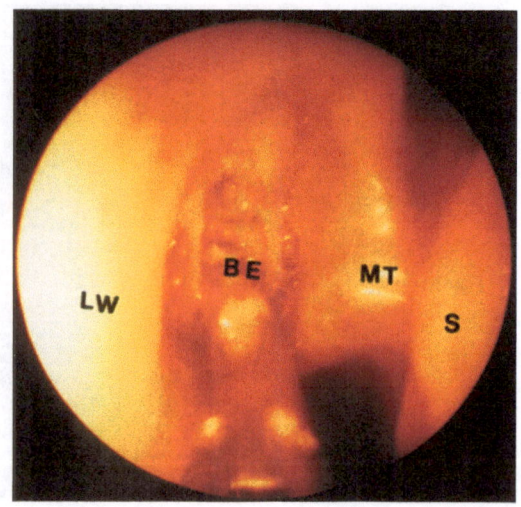

8.11

Fig. 8.8. **a** The incised uncinate process (UP) is grasped by means of an upward-cutting forceps at its superior and then its inferior ends, and mobilised gently medially, to detach it from the lateral nasal wall. **b** The intimate relations of the uncinate. LW, lateral wall; MT, middle turbinate; S, septum; O, orbit; FP, frontal process of maxilla; IT, inferior turbinate; MX, maxillary sinus; V, vomer; MC, maxillary crust; N, nasal bone.

Fig. 8.9. **a** Note the completely separated uncinate process (UP) from its superior to inferior ends, an infundibulotomy has been performed (polyps seen in the infundibulum). **b** Excised uncinate process with pneumatisation of its superior end. LW, lateral wall; P, polyp; MT, middle turbinate; S, septum.

Fig. 8.10. The initial incision must extend around the lower third of the uncinate process (UP), so as to expose the natural ostium (arrow). LW, lateral wall; MT, middle turbinate; S, septum.

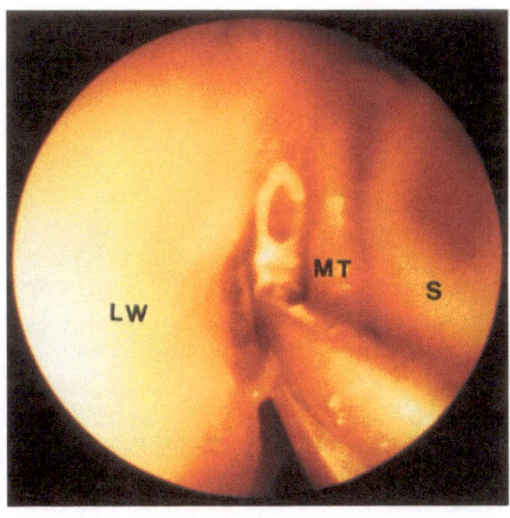

8.12

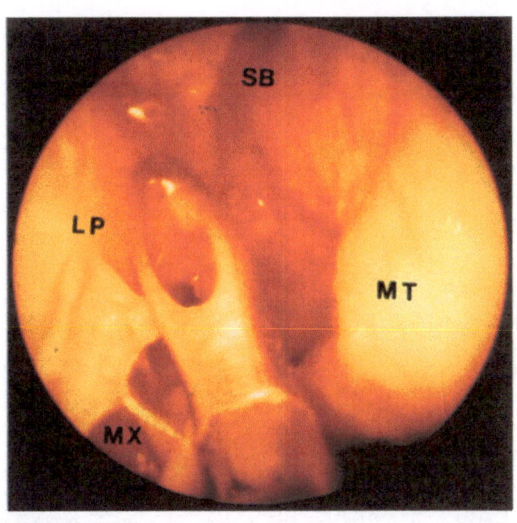

a

8.13

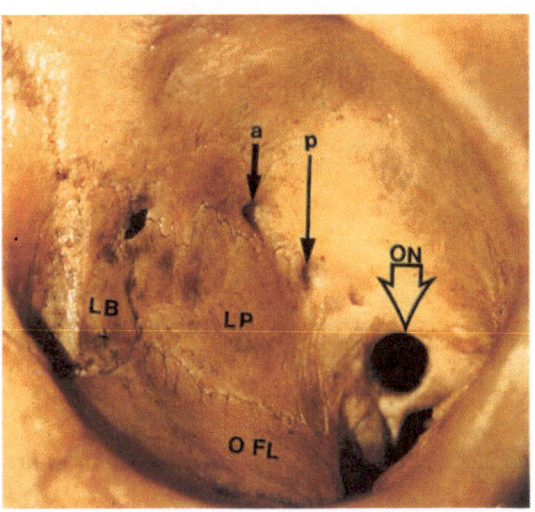

b

8.14

Fig. 8.11. Excision of the bulla, thus opening the middle ethmoidal cells. LW, lateral wall; BE, bulla ethmoidales; MT, middle turbinate; S, septum.

Fig. 8.12. Note the position of the forceps parallel to the lateral surface of the middle turbinate and lamina papyracea, with the middle turbinate constantly under vision. LW, lateral wall; MT, middle turbinate; S, septum.

Fig. 8.13. **a** Gentle removal of cells from the lamina papyracea. **b** The bony orbit showing ethmoidal arteries. a, anterior; p, posterior; ON, optic nerve; LP, lamina papyracea; SB, skull base; MT, middle turbinate; MX, maxillary sinus; LB, lacrimal bone; OFL, orbital floor.

Fig. 8.14. Identification of the skull base in the posterior aspects, note the olfactory nerves (arrow). OF, orbital fat (cadaver dissection). LP, lamina papyracea; SB, skull base; MT, middle turbinate.

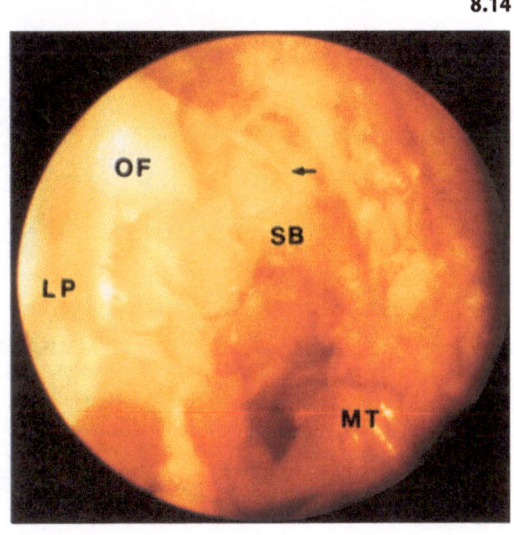

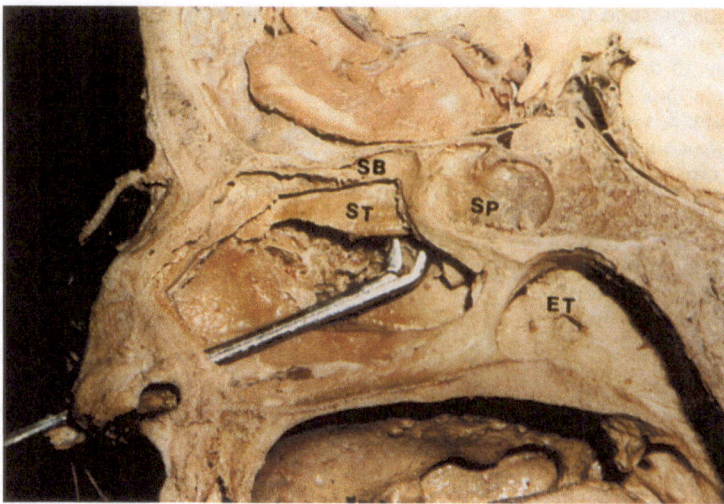

Fig. 8.15. Identification of the antero-inferior wall of the sphenoid sinus is important, so that its *infero-medial aspect* may be entered. SB, skull base; ST, superior turbinate; SP, sphenoidal sinus; ET, eustrachian tube.

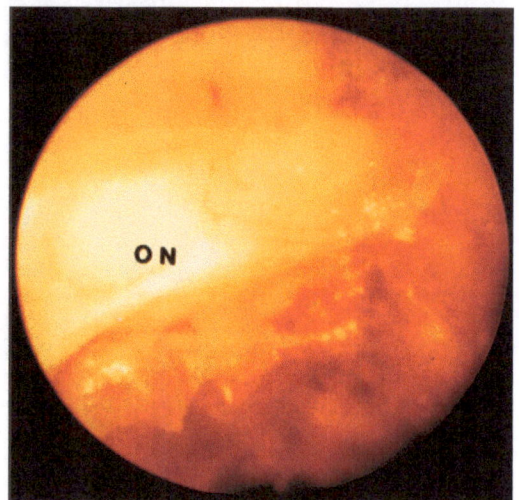

Fig. 8.16. The bulge of the optic nerve (ON) in the right sphenoid sinus.

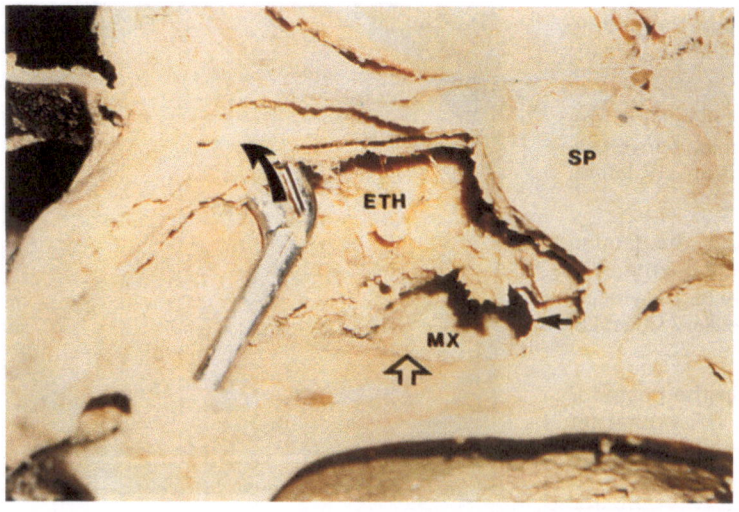

Fig. 8.17. After identifying the skull base posteriorly, dissection is carried out forwards to the frontal recess. ETH, excised ethmoid cells; MX, maxillary sinus; SP, sphenoid; arrow shows direction of frontal recess.

A sickle knife is used to carve out the uncinate process from its lateral attachment, from superior to inferior, and from anterior to posterior. The incision is parallel to the lateral border of the middle turbinate, and is taken in the groove usually seen on the lateral wall. The relation of the uncinate process to the orbit is of utmost importance: a laterally rotated process must be recognised on CT and tackled with due caution.

Uncinate Process

Inadequate removal of the upper part will lead to
1. difficulty in getting into frontal recess
2. may cause obstruction to the drainage of the frontal recess
3. adhesions may form which may obstruct frontal recess

Inadequate removal of the lower part will lead to
1. difficulty in getting into maxillary ostium
2. may cause obstruction of the infundibulum

Guidelines for Surgery

- meticulous atraumatic technique
- minimise bleeding – mucosal & arterial
- use 0° endoscope
- 30° and 70° 'scopes may cause distortion, trauma and bleeding
- identify landmarks: uncinate process/lamina papyracea/ground lamella/skull base
- approach should be directed medially and downwards as the endoscope is advanced

Operative Landmarks

- middle turbinate
- uncinate process
- lamina papyracea
- ground lamella
- skull base
- upper border of posterior choana
- anterior wall of sphenoid

The upward cutting (Weil–Blakely) forceps is used to grasp the uncinate process, and deliver it by gentle medial rotation by detaching superiorly and inferiorly. The base of the process is often left behind by beginners, leading to difficulties in identification of the natural os, and subsequent performance of an antrostomy. The uncinectomy allows a good view of the infundibulum, thus clearing the way for the next phase of the procedure.

The bulla (middle ethmoidal cell) is next removed using straight forceps. Careful dissection of the middle ethmoidal cells brings one to the roof of the ethmoid complex. The anterior ethmoid artery may be identified at this point, a useful landmark for the superior limit of the ethmoidectomy. The anterior ethmoid artery originates from the ophthalmic artery, a branch of the internal carotid system. It runs in a conduit along the skull base, and the junction of the middle and anterior ethmoidal cells. The medial limit of the dissection and the medial limit of the middle/anterior ethmoid complex is the upper attachment of the middle turbinate.

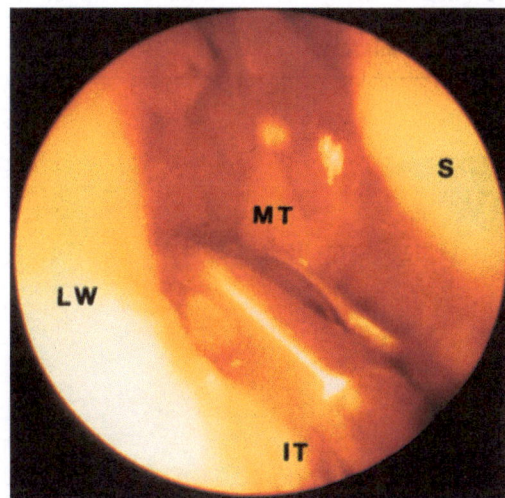

Fig. 8.18.   The first step for a middle meatal antrostomy is identification of the natural ostium at the lower border of the middle turbinate (MT) (if not already done). LW, lateral wall; IT, inferior turbinate; S, septum.

8.19

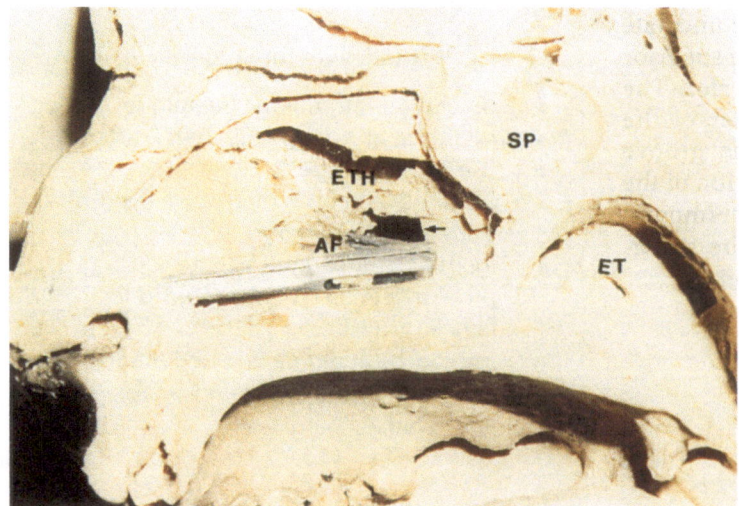

Fig. 8.19. The middle meatus is enlarged at the expense of the anterior fontanelle (AF) (antero-inferiorly). ETH, excised ethmoid cells; SP, sphenoid; ET, eutachian tube.

8.20

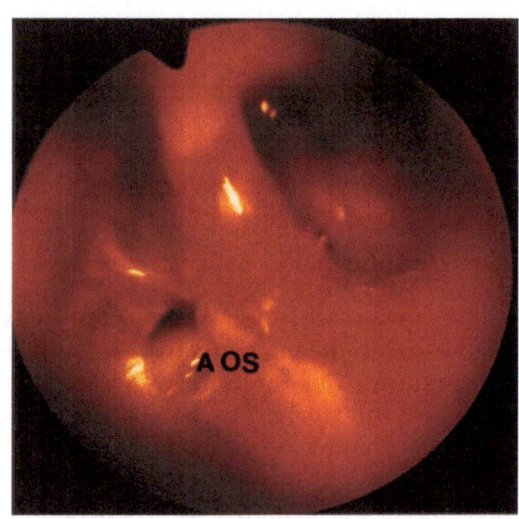

Fig. 8.20. To prevent recirculation of mucus, the natural ostium must be connected to an accessory one if present. Shown is an enlarged middle meatal antrostomy along with an accessory ostium AOS).

Fig. 8.21. **a** Wedge resection of MT, note approximately 0.5–1 cm of the anterior end of the middle turbinate is excised. **b** The excised wedge of the anterior end of the middle turbinate (MT), pneumatisation of the anterior end is seen. S, septum; LW, lateral wall.

8.21

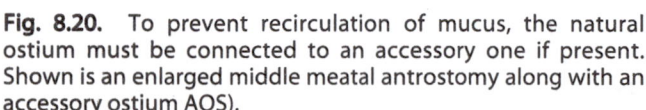

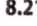

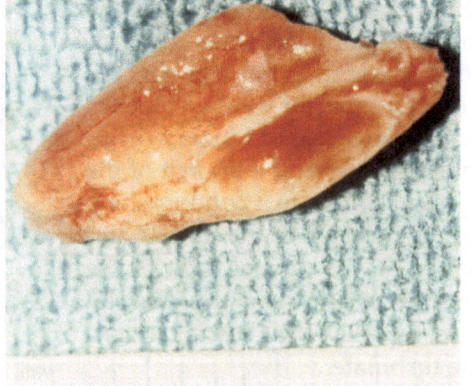

a

b

There is good reason to stay away from this superior junction of the middle turbinate with the skull base. The cribriform plate is thin here, and easily traumatised because of multiple perforations by the olfactory nerve. The ethmoid roof is hard throughout its length, but at its medial-most aspect it turns down sharply to join the cribriform plate, where it is quite thin.

The lamina papyracea is now identified, and kept in perspective throughout the operation. The ethmoid air cell complex is debulked gently, avoiding any tugging motions. All exenterated material is immersed in water to check for adipose tissue, a warning sign of breach of the lamina papyracea. Multiple small bites are better than a single large one. All forceps movements should be parallel to the lamina.

The skull base is identified posteriorly where it is at its thickest. The ground lamella is a thin plate of bone which connects the middle turbinate to the lamina paparycea. The perforation is always done medially to avoid traumatising the medial orbital wall. Once the larger posterior ethmoidal cells are identified, the endoscope should follow a gentle curve downwards and medially, *not upwards or laterally*. This prevents inadvertent entry into the cranium, or damage to the optic nerve.

If the posterior ethmoidal cells are seen to be clear, the procedure stops here. If, however, there is disease in this area, it is important to exenterate all cells with gentle biting movements from backwards to forwards. The antero-medial section of the roof is extremely thin; there is a distinct risk of breaching this boundary (danger area). Next the fourth important landmark is identified, the antero-inferior wall of the sphenoid sinus. This is opened and enlarged (sphenoidotomy). The sphenoid sinus is best opened at its inferior and medial aspect. The manoeuvre is carried out keeping in view the posterior choana which is 1 to 1.5 cm from the anterior sphenoidal wall. The sinus is normally at a distance of 7 cm from the anterior nasal spine. At 9 cm the tip of the forceps lies within the lumen. As a dehiscence of the internal carotid artery occurs in a quarter of patients, no instrumentation should be done within the sinus.

The middle meatal antrostomy follows, and we find that an incision along the caudal border of the uncinate process right up to the inferior end allows for better identification of the natural ostium. Landmarks locating the natural ostium are of crucial importance. The ostium usually lies at the same level as the inferior margin of the middle turbinate anterior to the bulla ethmoidales. Theoretically, the ostium is sited at the mid-point of the middle turbinate; however, this degree of depth perception is often difficult during an endoscopic procedure.

Finally, the close relationship of the ostium to the inferior orbital wall must always be kept in mind, and any evidence of lamina papyracea dehiscence must be looked for. The ostium is almost always in the same sagittal plane as the lamina papyracea, which by now should have been identified as a part of the ethmoidectomy. A helpful tip for identification of the os is the presence of air bubbles at the site. In difficult cases, as in gross sinus pathology, distorted anatomy or recurrent disease, we advise a trocar and cannula be passed through the inferior meatus into the sinus cavity, so that it may be irrigated under endoscopic vision. This helps to locate the position of the ostium. It should be remembered that fluid may exit the sinus through an accessory ostium as well, thus misleading the surgeon!

After identifying the ostium, it is denuded of its surrounding bone using upward-cutting forceps, and the antrostomy is now enlarged at

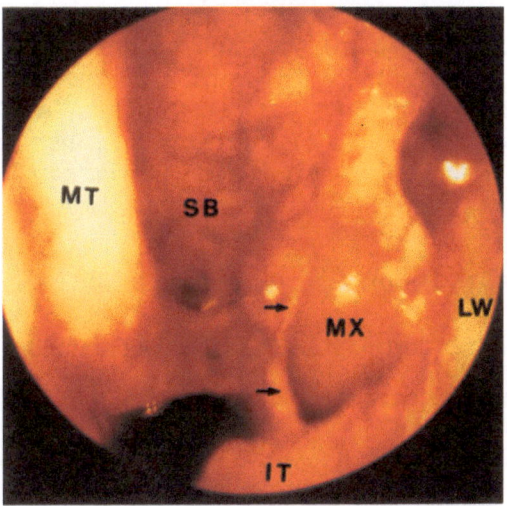

Fig. 8.22. Operated cavity as seen at the end of the procedure (left side). The arrows show mucosa everted over the antrostomy margin. MT, middle turbinate; SB, skull base; MX, maxillary sinus; LW, lateral wall; IT, inferior turbinate.

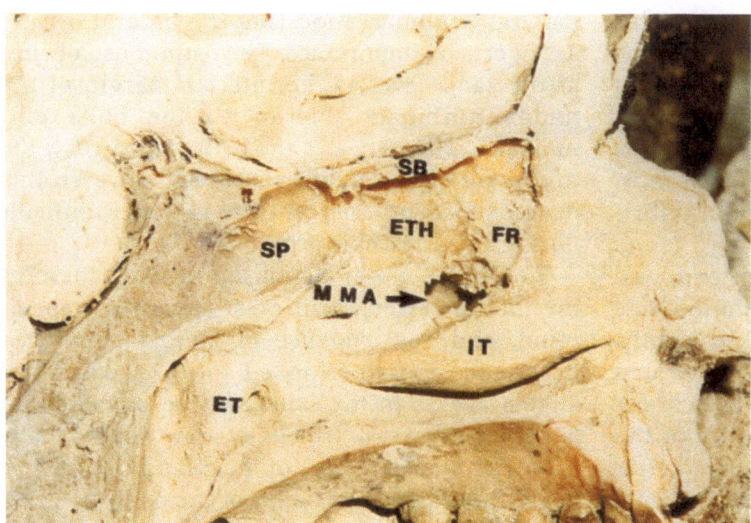

Fig. 8.23. Similar view to Fig. 8.22 in a cadaver. The relationship of the middle meatal antrostomy (MMA) to the inferior turbinate is seen. SP, sphenoid sinus; ET, eustachian tube; ETH, ethmoid canity; FR, frontal recess; IT, inferior turbinate; SB, skull base.

the expense of the antero-inferior fontanelle. A factor of paramount importance at this stage is that anterior sacrifice of bone must be stopped when the thickness of the fronto-nasal process of the maxilla is encountered or else unnecessary trauma may result in excessive bleeding. Also, the nasolacrimal duct may be damaged in this region, leading to epiphora in the post-operative period.

Differences between Accessory Os. & Natural Os	
Accessory ostium	**Natural ostium**
located in anterior and/or posterior fontanelle, sometimes multiple	located in the lower part of the infundibulum related to uncinate process anteriorly and bulla ethmoidales posteriorly
easy to identify	difficult to identify: can be found at the level of lower border of middle turbinate or upper border of inferior turbinate
circular or punched out appearance	usually oval-shaped
lies in saggital plane	lies more obliquely
present in 10% to 40% of patients	always present

Another tip concerns the opening itself; in order to prevent stenosis, it is prudent to "tuck in" the mucosa around the ostium as a final step.

Often the natural ostium is not easy to identify intra-nasally due to:

- thick periosteal bone
- scarring from prior surgery
- blood obscuring the operative field
- hypoplastic sinus
- gross pathology (polyposis)

In order to circumvent these problems, we employ a modified Messerklinger technique, combining intra-antral and intra-nasal views (CAMMA: Combined Approach Middle Meatal Antrostomy). Having exposed the ostio-meatal complex, a 0° endoscope is inserted through a sublabial cannula into the sinus, and the medial wall of the sinus is brought into view. Working through the nose with the other hand, the curved upward cutting forceps are used to enlarge the natural ostium. Since this is the only instrument in the nose at this time, the range of movements is quite free; in addition, the forceps teeth can be directly visualised through the endoscope as they gradually fashion the middle meatal antrostomy at the expense of the antero-inferior wall of the ostium. If an accessory ostium has been identified, it must be communicated with the natural ostium as a part of the middle meatal antrostomy.

The patient leaves the hospital after 24 hours if a concomitant operation such as septoplasty or

> #### Middle meatal antrostomy (infundibuloplasty): salient points
>
> **FACTS**
> - "MMA" is not synonymous with FESS!
> - a "hole" in the fontanelle is NOT "MMA"
> - a functional MMA is more important than the physical size of the MMA
>
> **Technique of MMA**
> 1. remove lower end of the uncinate process
> 2. preserve bulla ethmoidales until natural ostium is identified
> 3. remove stenotic areas of the ethmoid around natural ostium
> 4. remove any pathology around natural ostium with preservation of mucosa
> 5. connect natural ostium with the accessory ostium

septo-rhinoplasty has been performed. Patients operated on under a local anaesthetic are fit to go home the same evening, while FESS patients who have had a general anaesthetic go home the following day.

All in all, the CAMMA technique proves to be a safe method of visualising the natural ostium from within. It leaves the nasal cavity free for instrumentation, an important point for beginners who may find difficulty working in a limited space. The routine technique calls for three instruments (endoscope, cannula and forceps)

being passed into the nose simultaneously, each about 4 mm in diameter. The CAMMA procedure cuts this down to a minimum of one instrument. Furthermore, it is known that leaving a bridge of tissue between the natural and accessory ostia leads to a local recirculation of mucus and constant reinfection of the maxillary sinus. The technique permits direct visualisation of the ostia, thus facilitating their communication.

The final step is clearance of the frontal recess and agger nasi cells if there is disease in the frontal sinus. This is performed at a late stage in order to prevent soiling of the operative field by the almost certain oozing that takes place. For this procedure, a 30° or 70° 4 mm endoscope is recommended. Upward cutting forceps are used to enter the frontal recess at the attachment of the middle turbinate to the lateral wall of the nose. It is not always easy to find the frontal recess, as it may be surrounded by a cluster of anterior ethmoidal cells (agger nasi). However, in this situation, usually the *most medial cell* is the one which will lead into the frontal recess and ultimately into the frontal sinus.

We find exenteration of this rather inaccessible region is best performed by use of ophthalmic upward-cutting punch forceps. It is important to clear the anterior ethmoids, as one of the most common causes of recurrence and persistence of symptoms is the presence of disease in this region. Unfortunately, until adequate dexterity is achieved, one tends to overlook this part of the procedure as it is rather cumbersome working

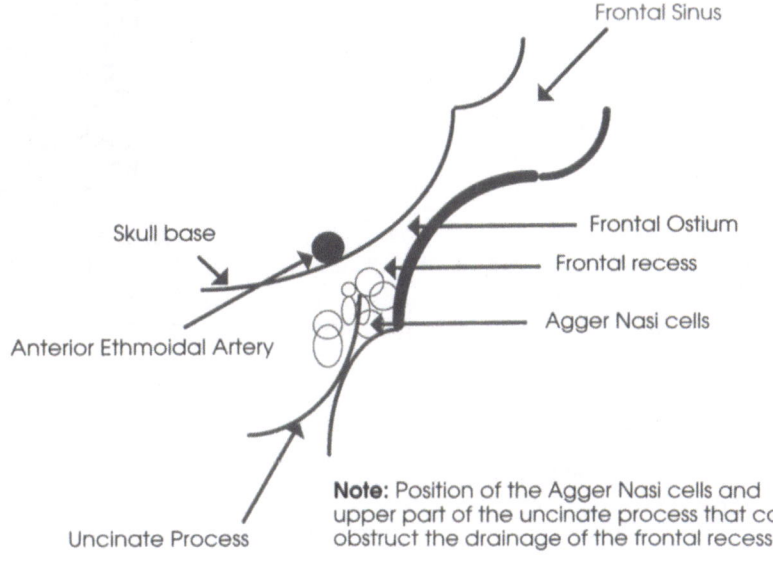

Fig. 8.24. Surgical anatomy of the frontal recess.

Note: Position of the Agger Nasi cells and upper part of the uncinate process that can obstruct the drainage of the frontal recess

through 30° and 70° endoscopes; however, it must be remembered that any compromise at this stage might well bring the patient back with residual disease.

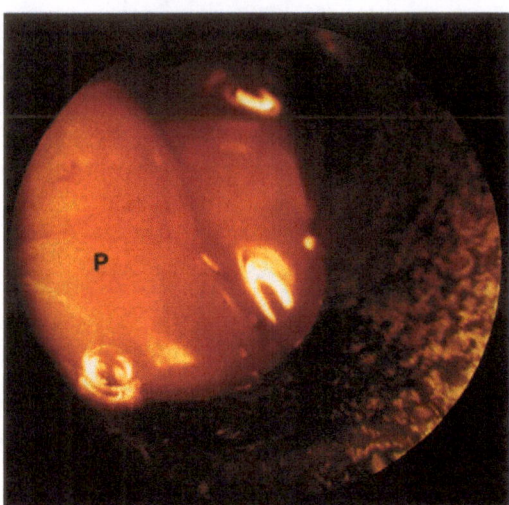

Fig. 8.25. Quite often, the maxillary sinus is full of thickened mucosa and polyps, and identification of the ostium is quite difficult. Not much is seen on antroscopy except polyp (P).

Surgery of the frontal recess

Difficulties

- Difficult surgical anatomy to understand on the operation table
- Dangerous area as it is close to skull base and orbit
- Surgical area is difficult to view
- 30° and 70° degree endoscopes need to be used. These endoscopes cause distortion and foreshortening of the surgical field and are difficult to handle
- Special instruments are needed
- It is extremely important to preserve the mucosa otherwise stenosis readily occurs
- Osteoneogenesis is common in this area
- Surgeon must learn the technique on cadavers

Key points in the surgical technique

1. Identify skull base and anterior ethmoidal artery
2. Use 30° and 70° degree endoscopes
3. Keep attachment of the middle turbinate and cribiform plate in sight all the time
4. Work in slightly lateral direction
5. Always work anteriorly
6. Never work anterior to posterior direction
7. Gently palpate with ostium seeker or suction cannula for "false" ceiling (egg shell consistency of the aggar nasi cells)
8. Always preserve mucosa
9. If stent is to be used never insert the stent tightly which may cause mucosal necrosis and stenosis

Anatomical relations of the aggar nasi cells

- Laterally: nasal and lacrimal bones
- Anteriorly: frontal process of maxilla
- Superiorly: frontal recess and frontal sinus
- Inferiorly and medially: uncinate process
- Posteriorly: ethmoidal infundibulum

Note: location and extent of pneumatisation vary widely

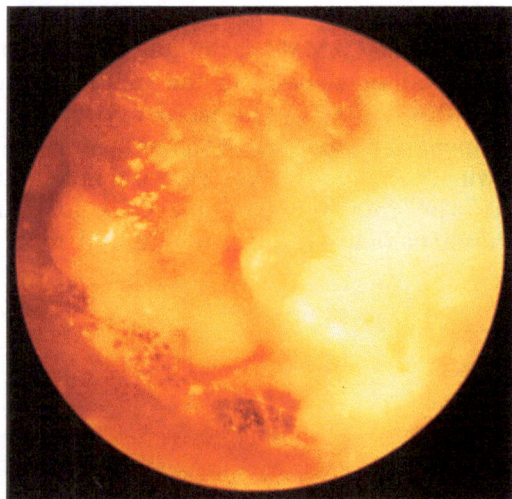

Fig. 8.26. Scarring, muco-pus or granulation tissue can obscure the view of maxillary natural ostium, as seen on antroscopy.

Fig. 8.27a–h. CAMMA technique. **a** Identify the canine fossa always lateral to the canine tooth. **b** A small stab is made through the mucous membrane. **c** The trocar and cannula are inserted through the canine fossa. **d** The endoscope is inserted through the sub-labial cannula into the sinus, while instrumentation is performed through the nose under direct vision. (From *Laryngoscope*, vol. 102, June 1992, with permission). **e** Backward cutting forceps seen enlarging the natural ostium under direct vision. P, polyps; PW, posterior wall of maxillary sinus. **f** Cysts may also be excised under direct vision. PW, posterior wall of maxillary sinus; c, cyst. **g** The sinus is irrigated, and outflow assesed through the nose endoscopically to check the size of newly fashioned antrostomy. **h** The stab incision may be closed with a single stitch.

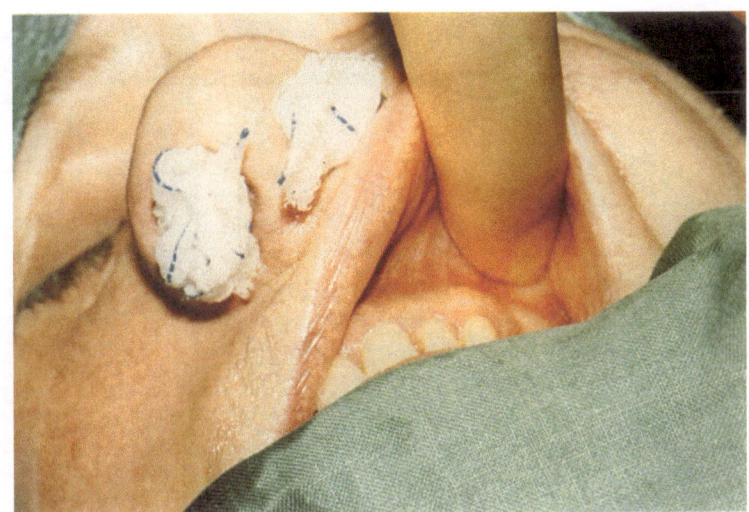

a

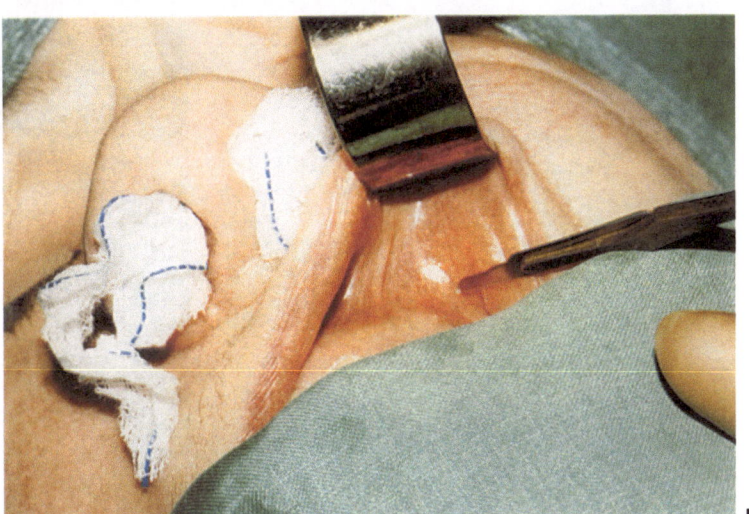

b

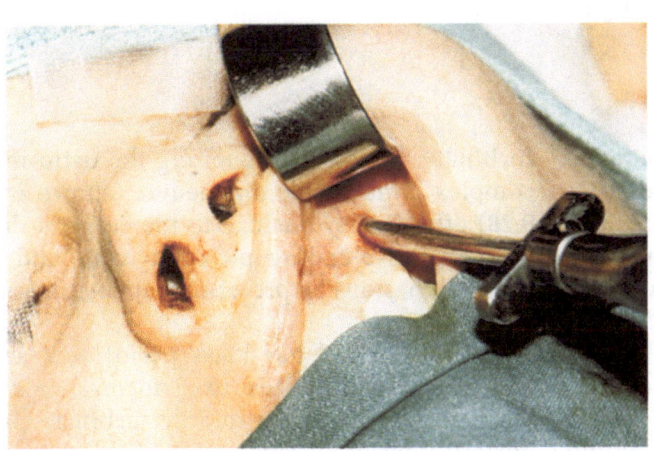

c

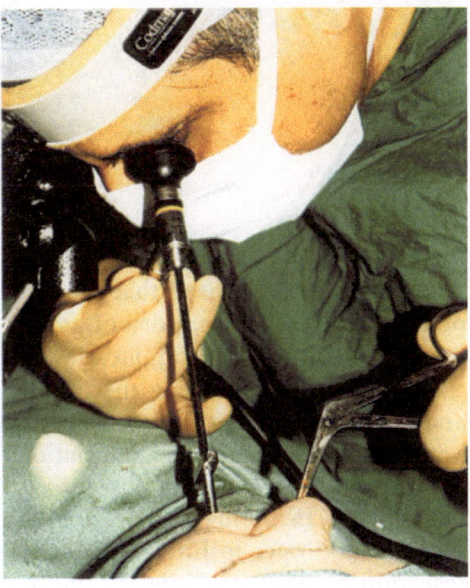

d

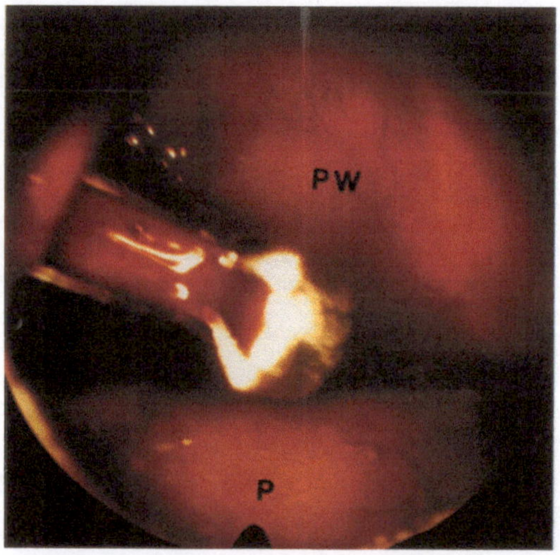

Fig. 8.27. *continued*

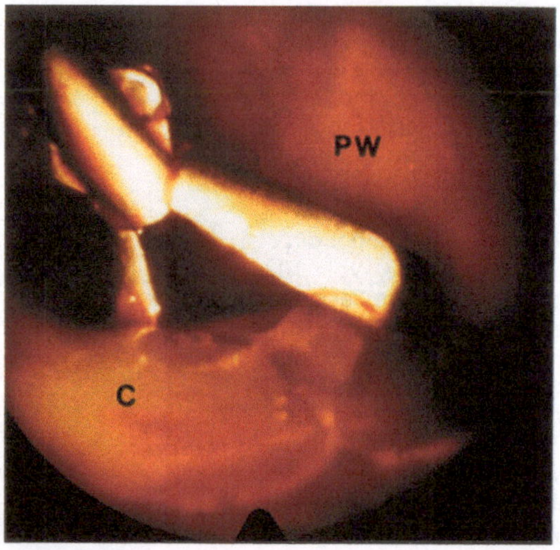

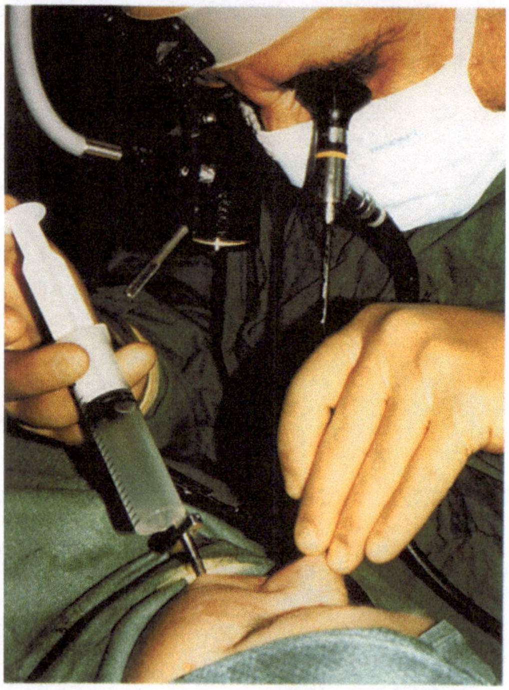

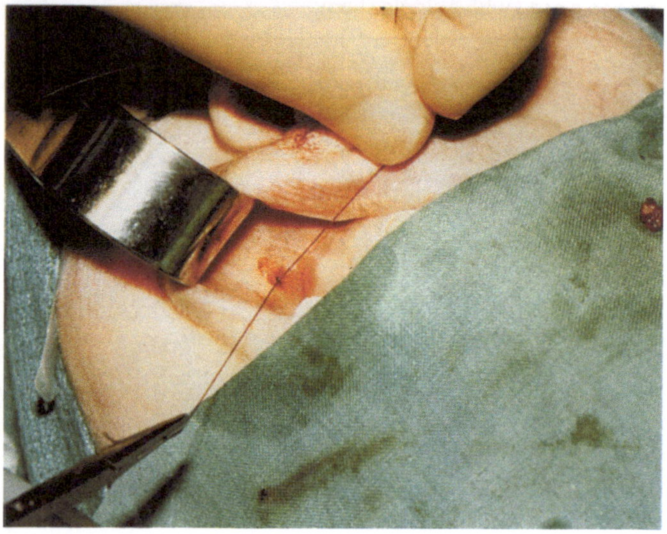

It is widely recognised that the post-operative period in FESS is as important as the operation itself. The commonest complication is the formation of adhesions between the middle turbinate and the lateral wall of the nose, which impede both mucous drainage and ventilation, as well as access to the operated field.

With this in mind, we have further modified the Messerklinger technique to include a wedge resection of the antero-inferior end of the middle turbinate, thus widely opening the ostio-meatal complex. This simple manoeuvre (shown in Fig. 8.28) affords easy passage to the surgeon during post-operative endoscopic cavity care, and minimises adhesions by preventing apposition of raw surfaces.

After the FESS has been performed, angled endoscopic scissors are used to make a cut in the anterior end of the middle turbinate (in the postero-inferior direction). A second cut joins the

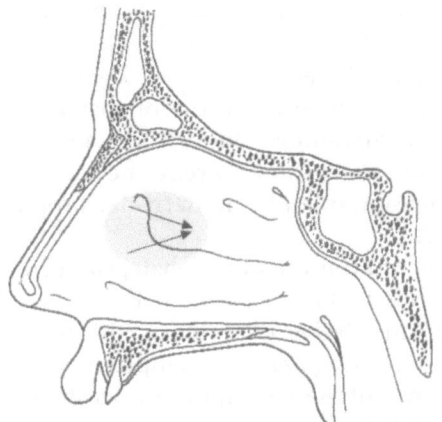

Fig. 8.28. Techniques of wedge resection of antero-inferior end of the middle turbinate. Upper arrow shows a cut in the posterior-inferior direction; lower arrow shows a cut in the infero-superior direction.

first from inferior to superior, thus freeing a small wedge approximately one sixth the length of the turbinate. Bleeding is usually minimal, and could be controlled by packing the nose for a few minutes. Under local anaesthetic, the procedure must be preceded by injection of lignocaine/adrenaline into the anterior end of the middle turbinate.

Our experience shows that significant number of middle turbinates do contain conchal cells, often showing mucosal thickening and/or pus, in spite of a radiologically normal turbinate on CT. It has been suggested that middle turbinate pathology may account for non-specific facial pains; this is borne out by our findings. Therefore, wedge resection also opens out an overt or latent concha bullosa.

Surgery of the Middle Turbinate

An enlarged middle turbinate due to either hypertrophied mucous membrane or to pneumatisation (concha bullosa) causes obstruction of the normal flow of air and/or mucus. Endoscopic visualisation under topical anaesthesia may reveal mucosal oedema in the middle meatus, but often there may be no overt evidence of disease. Plain films of the paranasal sinuses again do not aid in the diagnosis. On the other hand, CT is quite

effective in elucidating the extent of disease at an early stage. Additional findings such as mucosal swelling and blockage of the structures comprising the lateral nasal wall or ostio-meatal complex are often revealed (stenosis of the infundibular block).

Surgical management of a conchous middle turbinate must be based on its size and shape, and its relationship to surrounding structures (including areas of mucosal apposition). The nasal septum, the uncinate process and the anterior and middle ethmoidal sinuses all may be impinged upon by the turbinate laterally. If the septum itself is thickened superiorly, or is deviated towards the enlarged middle turbinate, it may be necessary to shave a wafer-thin layer off its cephalic cartilaginous portion and perpendicular plate by a septoplasty. Frequently, this itself improves nasal function. We excise the turbinate by wedge resection at its anterior end, as described earlier. In fact, a pilot study carried out by us revealed pus/polyps in middle turbinates that appeared otherwise normal, both endoscopically and radiologically. We now perform the procedure almost routinely. An attractive side-effect is the decrease in formation of adhesions between the lateral turbinate surface and the lateral nasal wall, although stringent post-operative care is still mandatory.

The Caldwell–Luc Procedure Revisited

The classical trans-buccal sino-rhinostomy operation was first described for the relief of chronic sinusitis by George Caldwell of New York in 1893. A few years later (1897), Luc in Paris proposed a similar technique. History bestowed the procedure with the combined names of Caldwell and Luc.

With the introduction of FESS, the traditional Caldwell–Luc procedure (CLP) has come under increasing scrutiny the world over. Long-term results evaluated at several centres indicate poor patient satisfaction, and persistence of disease as demonstrated by both endoscopy and CT. In fact, a large proportion of these patients have had to undergo FESS clearance. The reason for this is clear. The Caldwell–Luc technique involves accessing the maxillary sinus via the sublabial route, currettage of the sinus lining, and creation of an inferior meatal intra-nasal antrostomy. Thus the technique focuses only on exenteration of maxillary disease; furthermore, the inferior meatal antrostomy most often proves an inadequate answer to obstructive disease at the natural ostium. Today we know that the muco-ciliary pathways of the sinus are almost certainly genetically predetermined, and follow a route towards the natural middle meatal opening. Furthermore, chronic sinus disease almost always resides in the anterior ethmoids, which are not tackled at all during a CLP. Ironically, it was Caldwell who said, "the semilunar fold acts as an imperfect valve to the maxillary sinus, and incidentally guides fluids from the higher cells into the antrum, as I have repeatedly demonstrated on the cadaver. For this reason, the diagnosis of empyema of the antrum is not sufficient until the frontal and anterior ethmoid cells have been excluded. The antrum may be the *receptacle* (not the origin) of pus, or

become involved secondarily". This was as far back as 1893, the very year George Caldwell described the technique that bears his name. Restricted as he was with poor instrumentation, he was magnanimous enough to acknowledge his own limitations (and thereby the technique's), a fact often forgotten by modern-day proponents of the CLP.

In view of this ongoing debate, we reviewed our own series of 36 CLPs done over the last decade. In our cumulative experience, the incidence of persistent post-operative symptoms was 70%. A breakdown of these symptoms is as shown in Figs 8.29 and 8.30.

A fifth of these (20%) had patent antro-nasal windows at presentation. In the other cases (80%), the window was either completely occluded, or severely stenosed. Nasal endoscopy and CT scanning was performed, revealing an anterior ethmoid focus of disease *in all cases*. Our endoscopic findings ranged from common middle meatal obstructive factors such as turbinate para-

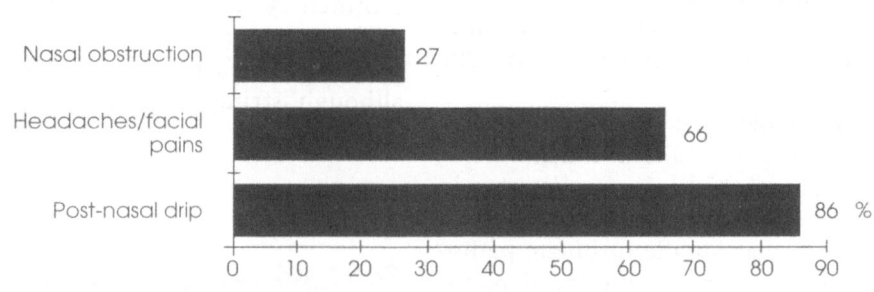

Fig. 8.29. Symptom profile of Caldwell–Luc patients (*n* = 36).

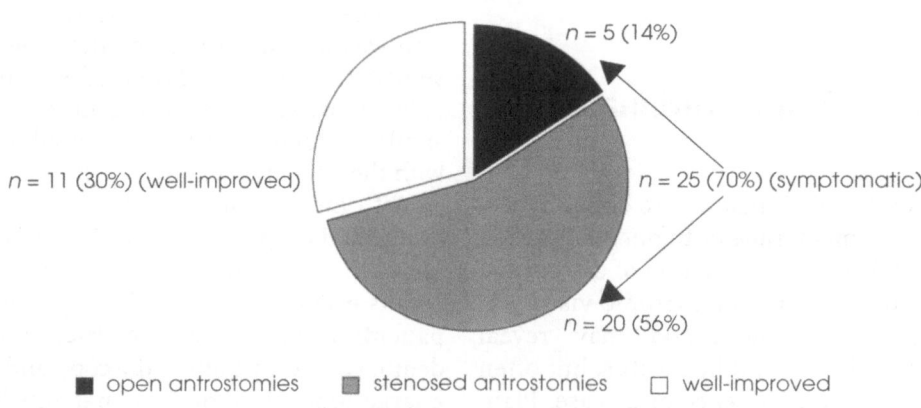

Fig. 8.30. Clinical findings of INA and outcome of our series of CLP patients.

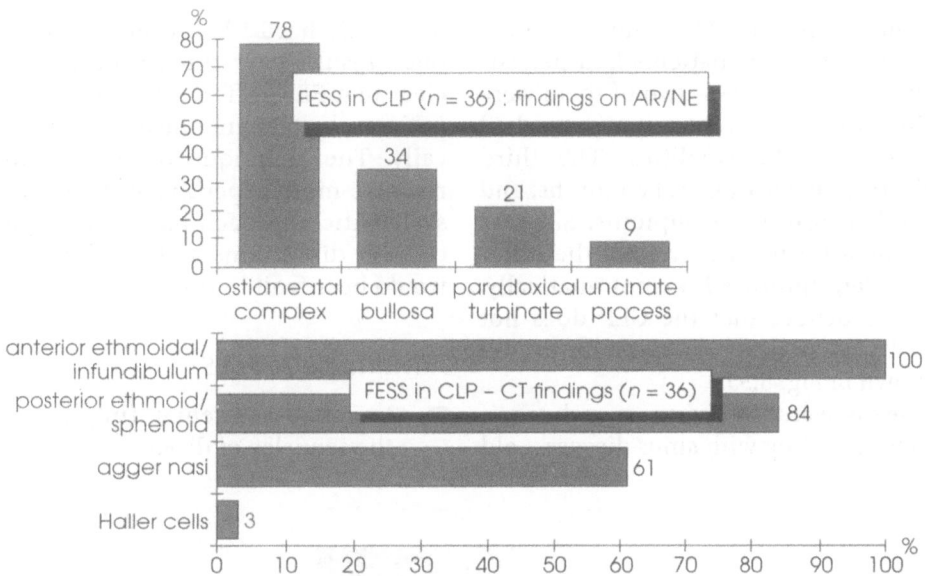

Fig. 8.31. Anterior rhinoscopy (AR), nasal endoscopic (NE) and CT findings in Caldwell–Luc patients (CLP) undergoing functional endoscopic sinus surgery (FESS).

doxicity, turbinate hyper-pneumatisation and medial/lateral rotation of the uncinate process to rarer turbinate malformations. CT confirmed endoscopic findings, and also showed anterior ethmoidal cell clouding and/or a narrow infundibulum, amongst other pathologies. These findings are displayed in Fig. 8.31.

As most studies so far have attempted to evaluate CLP results subjectively, we felt the need to develop an objective, easily performed, reproducible technique for CLP evaluation. Sterile saccharin was used to evaluate muco-ciliary clear-

ance time. In those cases where an the inferior meatal antrostomy was patent (open-window group), the solution was instilled through the antrostomy itself. In cases of stenosis or closure (closed-window group), the anterior fontanelle was used to access the sinus. Details of the actual technique may be found on page 18.

Our study confirmed that muco-ciliary timings were elevated in all of the 12 CLP patients examined, irrespective of the status of their antro-nasal windows. Pre-FESS times in this group averaged 50 minutes, while 6 month reviews revealed a

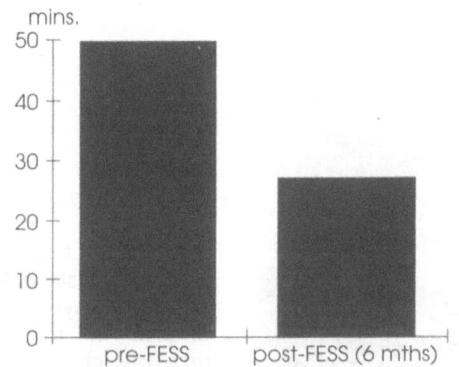

Fig. 8.32. Muco-ciliary clearence times.

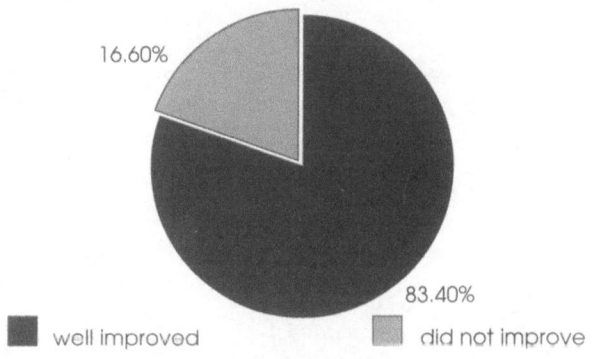

Fig. 8.33. FESS in CLP. Results after a follow-up of 9 months to 3 years (n = 36).

markedly reduced time of 27 minutes in nine patients (see above). Three patients had persistently delayed saccharin times – two of them were at 34 and 36 minutes – these might have had underlying mucosal abnormalities. The third showed no decrease in clearance at 6 months, and also had no relief from her symptoms. She was diagnosed to be aspirin-sensitive. All the other patients, however, improved symptomatically. This leads us to believe that the CLP does not control sinus disease in most patients. Our overall results are shown in Fig. 8.33.

No doubt one is averse to giving up such traditional methods of dealing with sinus disease – old habits die hard ! However, as one looks back at one's results over time, it becomes increasingly clear that FESS offers a better alternative to these patients, by tackling the disease more physiologically. The technique takes time to learn, and requires more expensive instruments; however, a systematic approach based on surgical anatomy, cadaver dissections and handling the endoscope would bear fruit in time.

Advantages of FESS

■ targetted at exenterating the cause and not the sequelae of disease

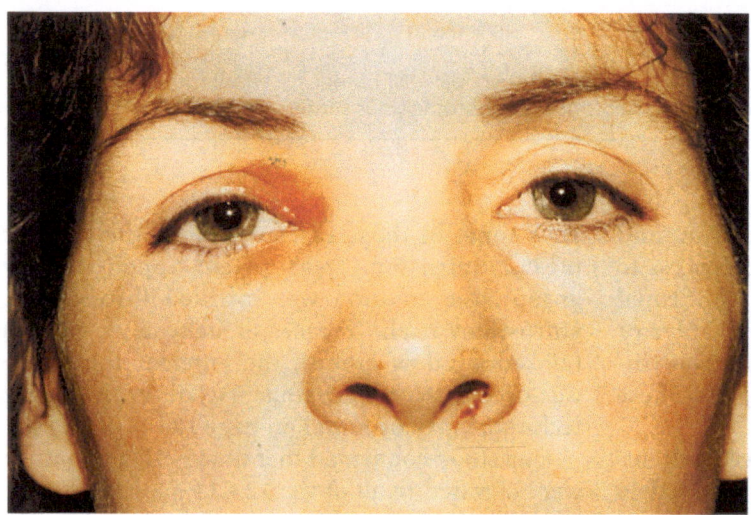

Fig. 8.34. If there is a dehiscence of the lamina papyracea, or a breach during the procedure, mild ecchymosis may result post-operatively, this settles in 3–4 days.

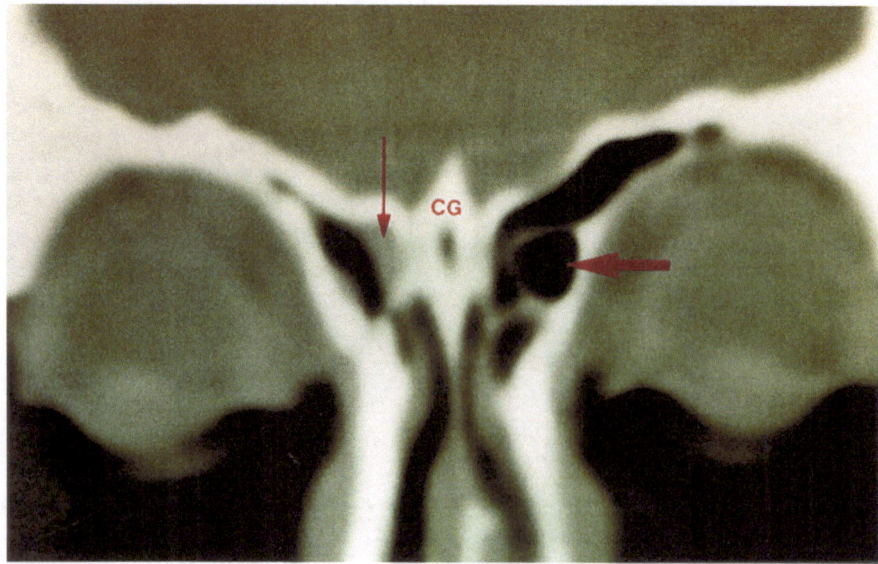

Fig. 8.35. Coronal CT scan. CG, crista galli; thin arrow shows mucosal disease in the frontal recess; thick arrow shows frontal cell obstructing frontal recess.

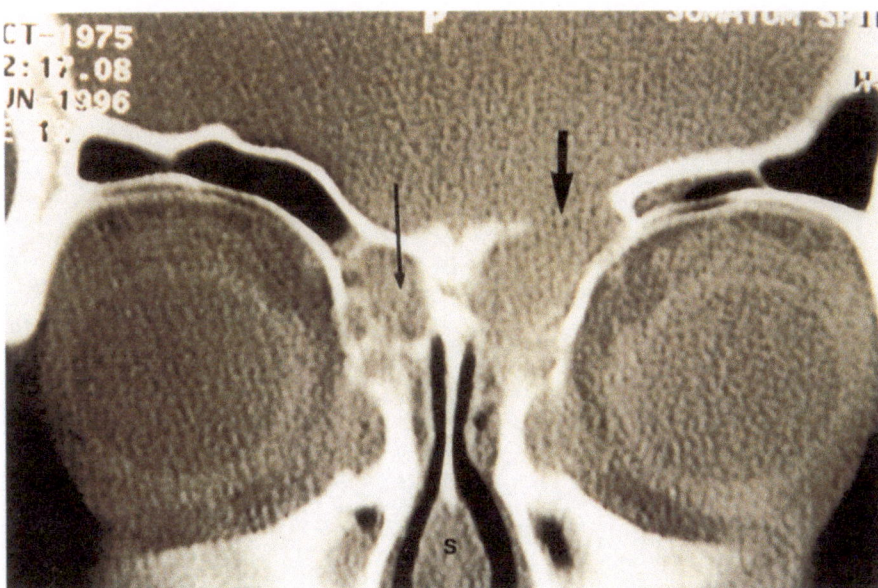

Fig. 8.36. Coronal CT scan showing bilateral frontal recess disease. Thin arrow shows mucosal disease in the frontal recess; thick arrow shows dehiscence of the superior wall.

- re-establishes normal ciliary function by drainage and ventilation of the sinuses
- can be performed under local anaesthesia on a day surgery basis and hence is cost-effective
- excellent visualisation of the operative area with multi-angled endoscopes

Disadvantages of FESS

- meticulous atraumatic technique is required for optimum results
- angulated endoscopes may cause disorientation, increasing the chances of complications
- use of endoscopes may give a false sense of security, the endoscope is not a substitute for surgical expertise but a useful tool
- because of the "microscopic view", the surgery may extend beyond required limits

Chapter 9

The Ethmoid Cavity: Post-Operative Care

The final ethmoid cavity is bounded by the lateral wall of the nose, the lamina papyracea, skull base and the middle turbinate. Posteriorly the cavity is related to the sphenoid, while antero-inferiorly it communicates with the nasal cavity. Into this space open the enlarged middle meatal antrostomy and the fronto-nasal recess. Thus the cavity acts as a portal for drainage from the maxillary and frontal sinuses.

It is of paramount importance to maintain the patency of the ethmoid cavity. We routinely apply ointment in the ethmoid cavity at the end of the operation (Soframycin/hydrocortisone). However, synaechia could remain a major problem in cavity care, leading to stasis, reinfection and poor surgical outcome. A correlation could be made between the mastoid and ethmoid cavity. Just as even a well-fashioned mastoid bowl requires assiduous toilet, an endoscopic ethmoidectomy must be regularly cleaned out until epithelialisation occurs.

The success of the procedure depends on meticulous care of the resultant ethmoid cavity. Nothing can replace regular follow-up till the cavity has healed satisfactorily. We see all post-operative patients in a special "Endoscopy Clinic". This is so that one might devote adequate time to their management, and a well-defined protocol could be established. Following discharge, the patient is seen twice-weekly for at least 2 weeks and weekly thereafter until the cavity begins to epithelialise. Every patient undergoing FESS with an instant septoplasty and/or rhinoplasty are advised to use warm alkaline nasal douch two or three times a day. Alkaline solution being mucolytic it also clears blood clots and crust from the the ethmoid cavity and enhances the epithelialisation. Our experience shows that this is very well tolerated by the patients as they tend to breathe more freely after nasal douch.

In endoscopic clinic the patient has his or her nose anaesthetised with 4% cocaine/adrenaline, and endoscopic suction clearance is performed. Blood clots, crusts, sequestrum and thickened mucosa are removed, as are small, residual polypi. The fibrous connections between the lateral wall and the turbinate are broken down, so as to prevent adhesions. Finally, the cavity is painted with an antibiotic/ steroid ointment. Post-operative antibiotics are not used routinely. They may be indicated if the procedure reveals extensive infection. In these cases, a broad-spectrum antibiotic is administered.

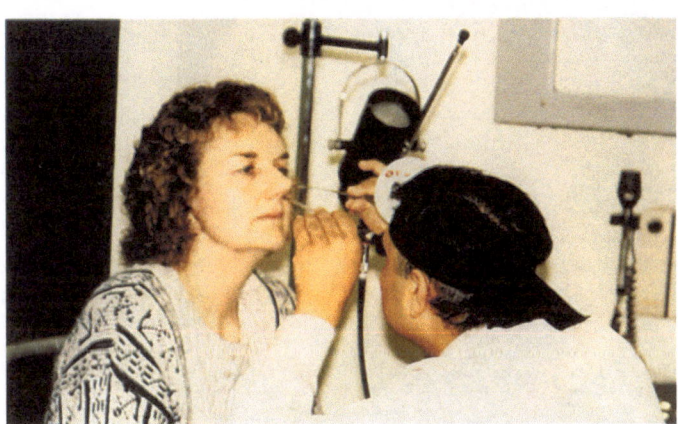

Fig. 9.1. The patient is seen in the endoscopy clinic after anaesthetic has been applied to the ethmoid cavity prior to endoscopic clearance.

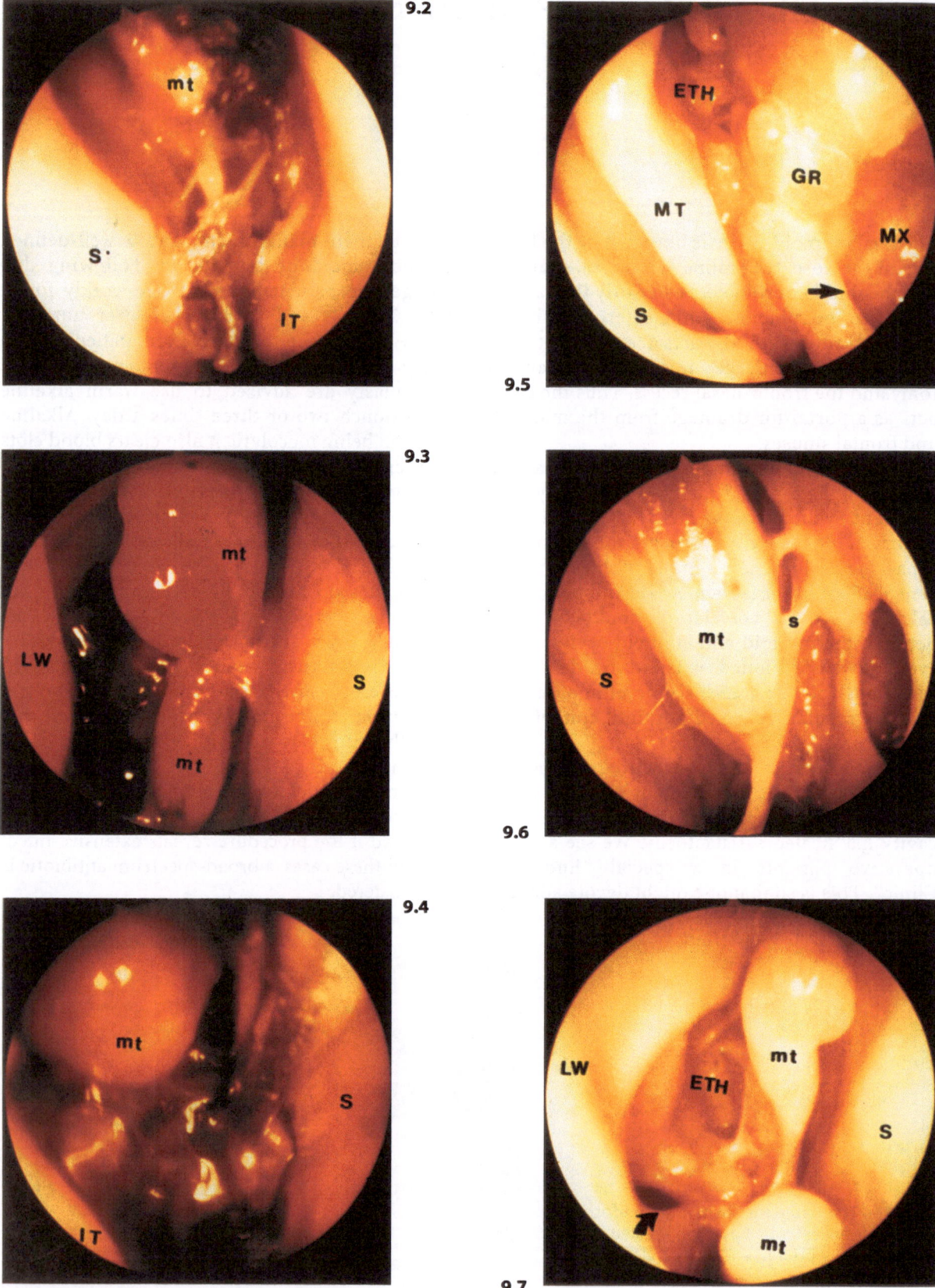

Fig. 9.2. Post-operative ethmoid cavity after 3 days, containing blood clots and crusts. Proper cavity care is essential. S, septum; MT, middle turbinate; IT, inferior turbinate.

Fig. 9.3. Wedge resection of the middle turbinate (MT) allows for proper access to the cavity (first post-operative week). LW, lateral wall; S, septum.

Fig. 9.4. Suction clearance of the ethmoid cavity, mucus and clots are removed. IT, inferior turbinate; MT, middle turbinate; S, septum.

Fig. 9.5. Four weeks post-operatively, note the granulations (GR) on the edge of the antrostomy (arrow), and in the maxillary sinus. This usually settles over a period of time. S, septum; MT, middle turbinate; MX, maxillary sinus; ETH, ethmoid cavity.

Fig. 9.6. Post-operative cavity after 6 months. Note small synaechiae (s), but large MMA with healthy sinus mucosa. S, septum; MT, middle turbinate.

Fig. 9.7. One year post-operatively, the ethmoid cavity (ETH) and MMA (arrow) are healthy. The unlocked ostio-meatal complex and ethmoid cavity are seen. LW, lateral wall; MT, middle turbinate; S, septum.

Fig. 9.8. Three years post-operatively, a small adhesion (A) has formed over the MMA (arrow); however, the cavity is clear. A small retention cyst (C) is noted. ETH, ethmoid cavity; S, septum.

Fig. 9.9. A classical MMA (small arrow) and widened frontal recess (curved arrow) at 4 years is the result of meticulous follow-up. MT, middle turbinate; MX, maxillary sinus.

Fig. 9.10. If care is not exercised, adhesions would form as shown. LW, lateral wall; MT, middle turbinate; S, septum.

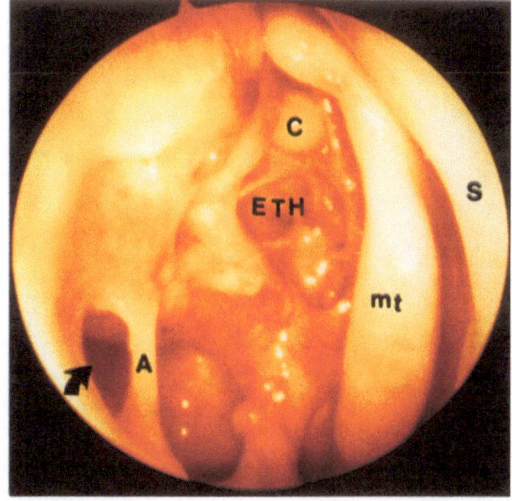

9.8

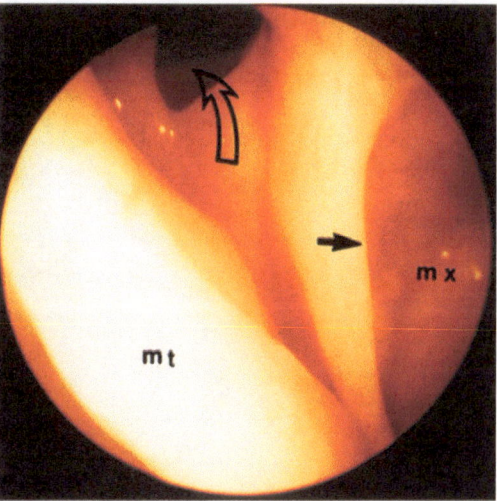

9.9

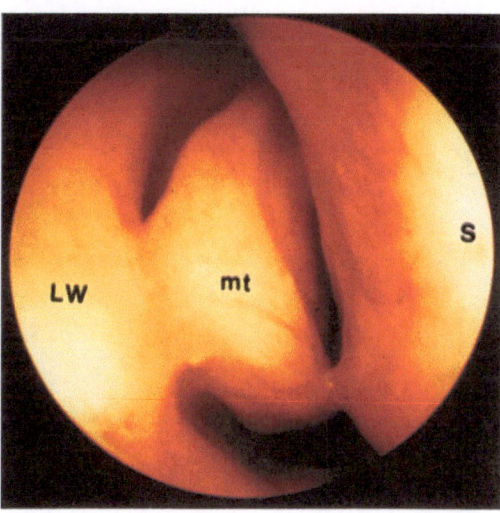

9.10

Chapter 10

Headaches and Facial Pains

Sinus disease almost always starts in the middle meatus. Both secretion and ventilation have to take place through the very narrow infundibular isthmus. Any narrowing or blocking of these spaces may lead to retention of secretions and/or poor ventilation, thus predisposing to chronic infection. At times, localised areas of contact of apposing mucosal surfaces in the key areas of the anterior ethmoids may lead to such a blockage and alter nasal function. Ciliary beating stops at the site of mucous membrane contact, thus causing stasis and providing ideal conditions for viral and bacterial infections. These localised mucosal factors may be summarised as

- constant intense mucosal contact
- poor ventilation or non-ventilation of the sinus with resulting hypoxia
- pressure from proliferating polyps

The sinuses may cause pain by the following mechanisms:

- Mechanical, due to blockage of sinus ostia. Here, the pain is poorly localised to the areas of Vth nerve distribution. It may vary in degree. Wolf (1955) has shown that the mucous membrane of the nose and sinuses has varying degrees of sensitivity, so that stimulation of the turbinates causes the least amount of pain, while instrumentation of the frontal recess causes moderate pain. The sinus ostia produce severe pain on stimulation. The two main stimuli that cause pain are temperature and pressure, so that even a slight touch with cotton wool in the region of the ostium could cause severe pain.

- Functional, due to affection of cilia, and mucosal oedema. Precipitating factors include exotoxin producing organisms and nasal irritants (e.g. noxious fumes) and allergens (e.g. pollens).

The occurrence of headaches and facial pains as a result of inflammation of the mucous membrane of the nose and sinuses in acute sinusitis is well known. In this situation, there is a blockage of the natural ostium, retention of secretions and mucosal irritation leading to hypoxia and a sensation of pain in the distribution of the Vth nerve. Furthermore, Stammberger (1988) also showed that negative pressure due to malventilation leads to bleeding into the infected sinus, and initiates pain. With the development of multi-angled endoscopes, it is now possible to explore the clefts of the nasal cavity, and to assess various structures in the region of the ostio-meatal complex. For example, areas of mucosal contact between two apposing surfaces lead to ciliary stasis and changes in the microvascular supply, causing reflex engorgement of the tissues and thus chronic inflammation and local increase in the concentration of vasoactive amines. These vasoactive amines are potent biotransmitters such as noradrenaline and acetylcholine; these act by inducing pain, or lowering pain threshold. They also reach blood vessels, and affect nasal secretions. Uddman et al. (1983) discovered a further transmitter, substance P. This is another potent neurotransmitter for sensory neurons, which acts locally in nasal mucosa as a strong vasodilator, and induces plasma extravasation, hypersecretion and smooth muscle contraction (this may account for the lower respiratory tract symptoms). Substance P further triggers oedema by simultaneous release of histamine from the mast cells.

Two further kinins exist in the submucosa of the nasal mucous membrane around blood vessels and glands. These are tachykinins and neurokinins. These also co-exist with substance P in C fibres, which carry the sensation of pain.

The work of Aust and Drettner (1974a) implicates three sinus factors in the production of pain: the size of the ostium, the sinus volume and the degree of nasal breathing. Functional sinus ostial size is directly proportional to oxygen exchange, while sinus volume is inversely proportional. This means that a small change in the diameter of the ostium, such as that due to mucosal thickening or blockage by polyps, has a dramatic effect on the exchange of oxygen in the maxillary sinus. Furthermore, oxygen exchange is twice as fast during nasal respiration as it is with the nostrils closed.

In all cases of possible sinus pain, a differential diagnosis must be kept in mind:

- Temporo-mandibular dysfunction
- tension headaches
- migraine
- brain tumours
- post-head injury (including whiplash)
- cervical arthritis
- neuralgias

CT scanning enables us to discover disease otherwise hidden from the eye. Some of the typical and more frequent abnormalities predisposing to headaches and/or recurrent sinusitis are listed in Table 10.1.

Table 10.1. Abnormalities predisposing to headaches and/or recurrent sinusitis

Septal abnormalities	Ethmoidal labryrinth	Uncinate process
High deviated nasal septum	Agger nasi cells	Medial rotation
Spur onto ostio-meatal complex	Middle turbinate concha bullosa paradoxical turbinate	Lateral rotation
		Contact with middle turbinate
Apposition of septum to superior turbinate	Large ethmoid bulla filling middle meatus	Pneumatisation
	Mucosal apposition	

A detailed analysis of clinical findings on anterior rhinoscopy and nasal endoscopy is shown in Fig. 10.1.

Not all these conditions are disease states *per se*, but they are factors that may reduce the already narrow spaces of the anterior ethmoids, and thus give rise to areas of mucosal contact, secretion retention and poor ventilation, and/or infection of larger sinuses. This promotes polypoid regeneration of apposing mucosal surfaces.

Key Points

- sinus pathophysiology as a cause of headaches and facial pains is well established
- "headache" patients must undergo a thorough nasal endoscopic examination
- CT findings such as concha bullosa, large bulla ethmoidales and a crowded ostio-meatal complex in conjunction with history and endoscopy are indications for surgery
- Endoscopic sinus surgery is the treatment of choice in such patients
- *The nose and sinus should be considered as one functional unit*

All these conditions, even when very small and circumscribed, may have one dominating clinical symptom of headache.

Coronal CT scanning was performed in all cases; it confirmed the clinical findings seen above. In addition, Fig. 10.2 shows disease in the agger nasi and Haller cells; 10% of our CT's were reported as normal, no mucoperiosteal thickening was noted.

The character of conchal pain is described as intermittent, and is said to be due to cyclic congestion of the lining mucous membrane. As a result of inflammation, a swelling of the middle turbinate presses on to surrounding structures such as the septum, producing pain over the medial canthus, the supraorbital region and occasionally the side of the face. The pain is mediated via branches of cranial nerve V2, and via peripheral interconnections with V1. Such headaches, unlike migraines, are not associated with auras, and may often occur in a dry nose. Moreover, they are of considerably shorter duration than migrainous headaches, and respond well to vasoconstrictor agents. The diagnosis is made from the character of the pain, and is confirmed by immediate relief with the application of a vasoconstrictor to the points of contact between septum and the lateral nasal wall. These contact points should be further evaluated by a coronal CT scan.

In keeping with these concepts, we analysed our data of 60 patients who presented with headaches and/or facial pains as a *predominant* feature. They ranged in age from 16 to 54 years (average age 34 years). The male to female ratio was 32 : 28, and follow-up extended from 8 months to 6 years.

The results are shown in Fig. 10.3.

As can be seen from Fig. 10.3, the majority of patients were well improved (very pleased with results) or improved (with intermittent symptoms, 52 in all). We do not know why eight patients did not do well.

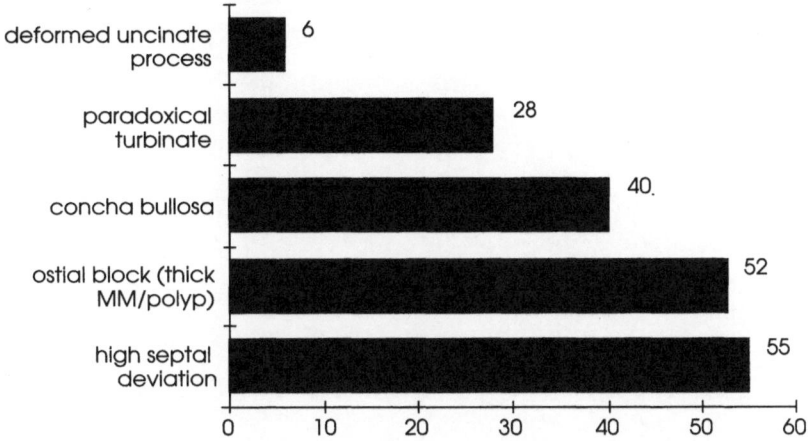

Fig. 10.1.   Clinical findings on anterior rhinoscopy and nasal endoscopy in 60 patients. Figures given are percentages.

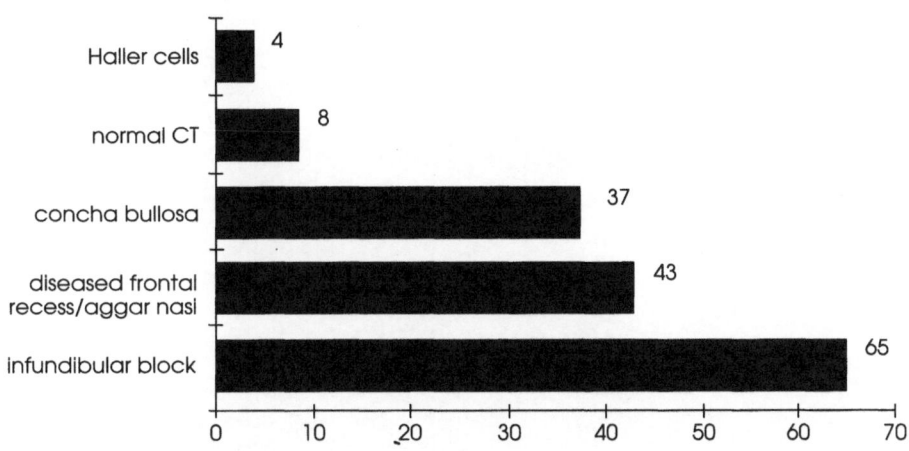

Fig. 10.2.   Findings on CT scan in 60 patients. Figures given are percentages.

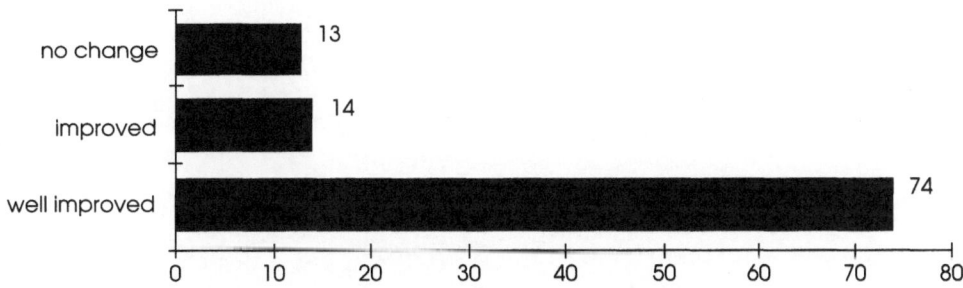

Fig. 10.3.   Results of FESS in treating headaches and facial pains in 60 patients. Figures given are percentages.

Chapter 11

Complications in FESS

Complications in FESS take on special significance, as a minimal indiscretion or breach of surgical landmarks may result in severe morbidity including intra-orbital and intra-cranial complications. Nowhere is the axiom "prevention is better than cure" more valid than in this intricately contoured region. Careful training and planning are vital to a successful outcome. We have classified the complications as described in Fig. 11.1.

The most troublesome complication during surgery is *bleeding*. Usually it is not severe enough to cause the procedure to be abandoned, but therein lies the danger, the surgeon proceeds with compromised vision, making his task more difficult, and risking complications. Bleeding may occur from one of two sources: a generalised mucosal ooze due to clumsy instrumentation, or a brisk, arterial bleed due to injury to the anterior or posterior ethmoidals, or branches of the spheno-palatine artery, packing usually controls the bleeding. The posterior septal artery, which supplies the posterior middle turbinate and septum, can bleed vigorously, and is controlled with cautery and packing. If the patient has had a recent insult to his respiratory lining by an upper respiratory tract infection, it is wise to institute a course of systemic antibiotics and decongestants before taking him up for surgery. Bleeding diatheses must be excluded, and it is important to note that patients with aspirin intolerance often exhibit an increased clotting time.

Pre-operative nasal packing must be gentle, it is often at this stage that an impatient surgeon sets off a potential problem. We "walk our pack in", i.e. starting anteriorly within the nasal vestibule, several packs are placed sequentially, towards and finally into the middle meatus. In addition, a pack is compactly positioned against the roof of the nasal cavity, thus desensitising branches of the ethmoidal nerves. We recommend cotton wool strips or soft universal strips instead of ribbon gauze. An average of five strips are used on each side, each staying in place for several minutes.

Vessel trauma poses a more serious threat to the procedure, if only because ligation or even coagulation is impossible. Packing and waiting is the rather frustating answer. The danger point for anterior ethmoidal damage during FESS is when the sinus lateralis is entered above the ethmoid

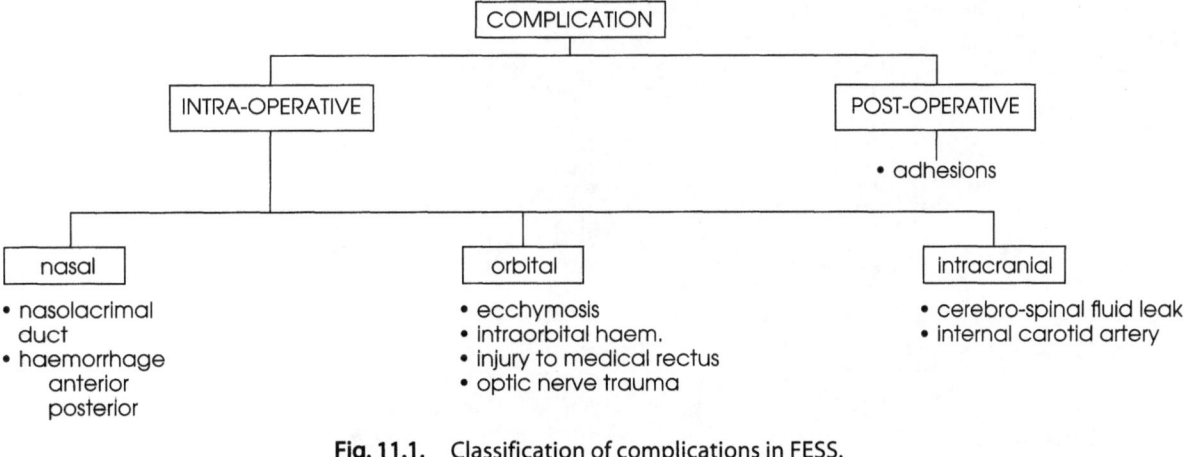

Fig. 11.1. Classification of complications in FESS.

bulla. It is here that the artery is seen to arch across from the lamina papyracea into the ethmoidal cells. The posterior ethmoidal is sometimes encountered after entering the ground lamella, especially if the endoscope is not forwarded in a parabolic fashion. Of the sphenopalatine artery, it may be said "the last, but most certainly not the least". As it exits the sphenopalatine foramen, it divides to supply the lateral wall of the nose. The anterior branch may be grasped and injured while enlarging the posterior limits of the middle meatal antrostomy. In addition, a mild *peri-orbital ecchymosis* may occur with compromise of the lamina papyracea, either due to the surgeon, or due to inherent dehiscence.

The opening of the *naso-lacrimal duct* is securely tucked away under the inferior turbinate, and rarely enters the surgical field. However, while resecting the anterior fontanelle with the backward-cutting forceps, there is a distinct risk to the duct, which lies only a few millimetres away. This is especially important in children. It is prudent to stop as soon as thick bone is encountered. Post-operatively if the patient develops epiphorae, an ophthalmologist's opinion should be requested.

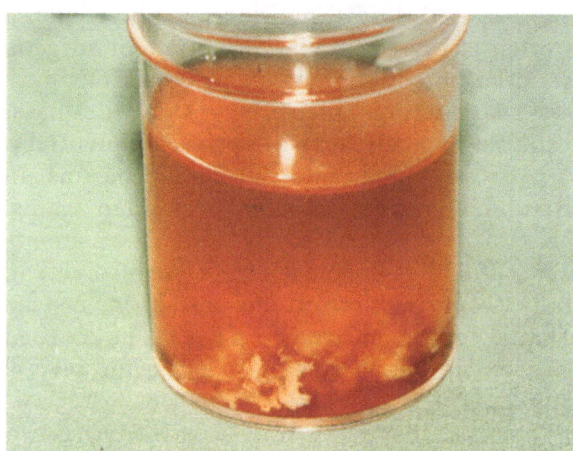

11.2

Fig. 11.2. Place all material removed from the ethmoid cavity into water, it must sink, only fat and brain tissue does not.

Fig. 11.3. In case of any doubt as regards breach of the lamina, gentle pressure should be applied to the eyeball to see the transmitted movements through the endoscope, and caution exercised.

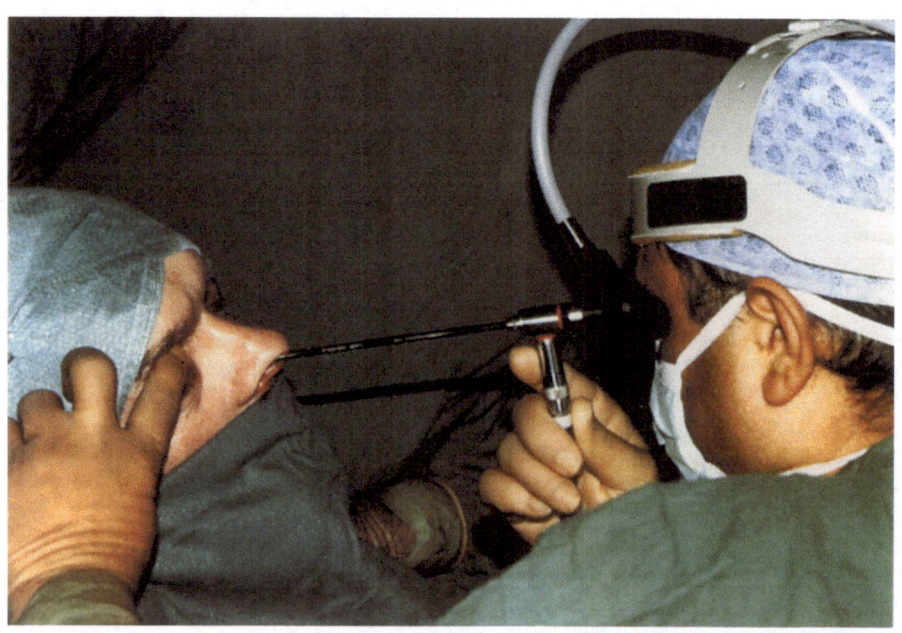

11.3

11.4

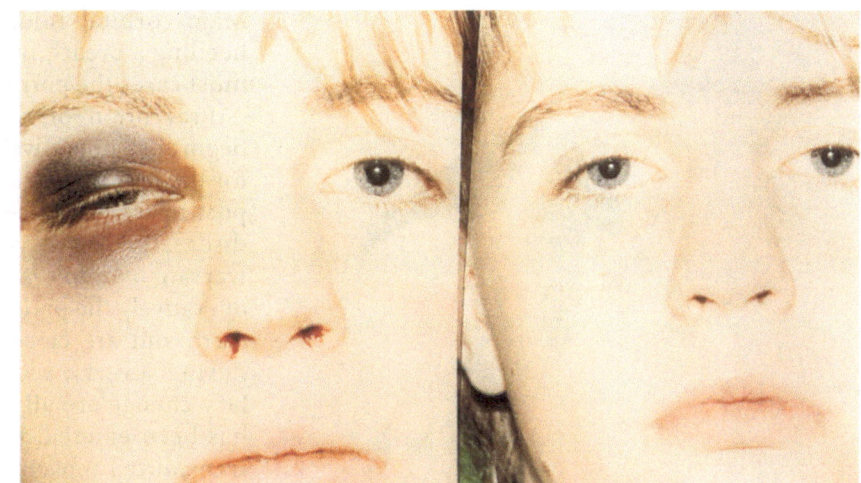

Fig. 11.4. With exposure of the orbital periosteum, a mild ecchymosis may occur in the immediate post-operative period – close observation must be maintained. The ecchymosis settles in 3 to 4 days.

Fig. 11.5. Patients should be instructed not to blow their noses for several days, as this may lead to a surgical emphysema (around the orbit on the right, arrow). Again, this settles rapidly.

Fig. 11.6. Acute sinusitis causing intra-orbital complications such as cellulitis and/or abscess should be treated endoscopically only by the experienced surgeon; otherwise conventional methods are employed.

Fig. 11.7. The same patient post-operatively.

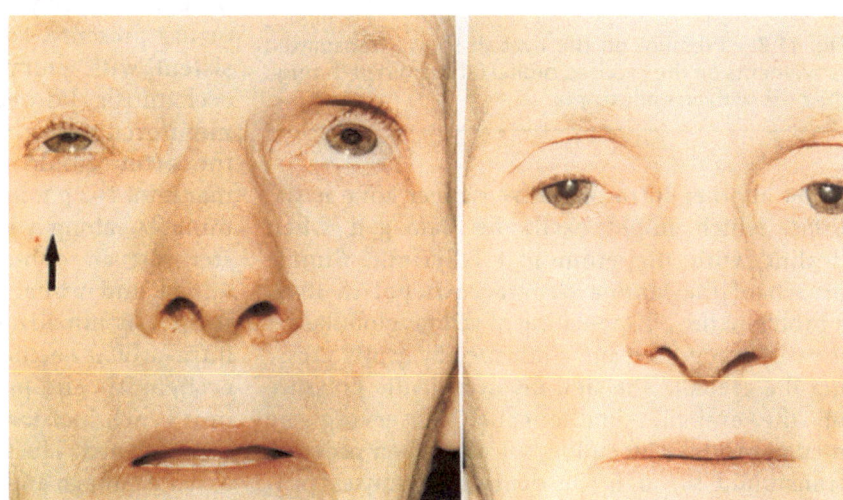

11.5

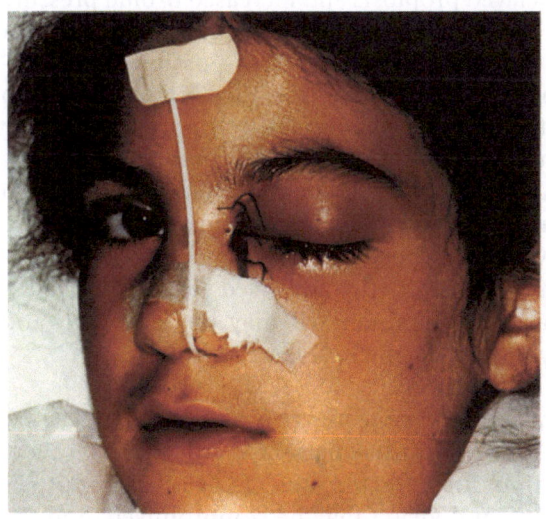

11.6

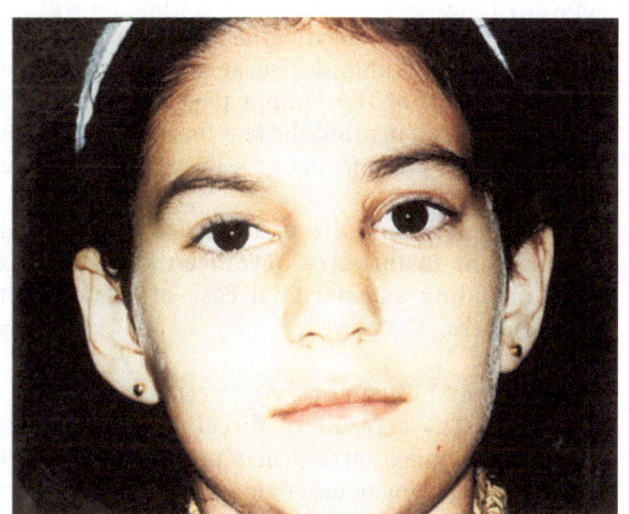

11.7

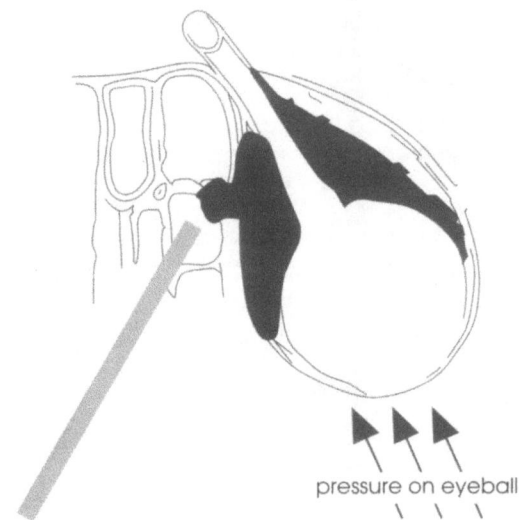

Fig. 11.8. Pressure on the eyeball shows transmitted movements on the exposed orbital fat examined through the nose with an endoscope.

Yet another intra-operative danger zone is the *orbit*, which might easily be damaged when dealing with the ethmoidal labyrinth. Simple breach of the lamina papyracea is not in itself a problem; the out-pouching of yellow, globular fat is easily recognised and confirmed by gently pressing the eyeball. The sign involves gentle pressure on the eyeball, simultaneously observing the medial orbital wall endoscopically, when pressure transmitted through the dehiscence causes protrusion of orbital fat into nasal cavity. (Fig 11.8)

Another simple check is to immerse all endoscopically removed tissue into water, when fat will be seen to float, thus alerting the surgeon to possible danger. As ethmoid disease is exenterated from the region of the lamina papyracea, it is important to keep in mind the fact that the lamina lies in the same plane (more or less) as the lateral wall of the nose.

Unfortunately, in spite of careful technique, complications in this area have been known to occur, including an anecdotal case of bilateral total blindness.

Blindness may be temporary or permanent, the latter occurs as a result of direct optic nerve injury or prolonged intra-ocular pressure due to haematoma, causing neural damage. Direct injury to the optic nerve is irreversible, whereas increased intra-ocular pressure could be reversed.

Major orbital injury occurs as a result of not heeding a breach in the lamina papyracea, and in most cases the peri-orbita too.

Prevention of this catastrophic complication begins pre-operatively, when evaluating the patient for the first time, and carries over to operative and post-operative phases. Patients who have extensive disease and/or have had previous interventions warrant caution and careful evaluation. Intra-operatively the patient's eyes are always left uncovered, and are closely observed. Eye movements during surgery, ecchymosis, proptosis and pupillary change are all signs which indicate the orbit has been entered. If pressure on the eyeball with transmitted movements is encountered with protrusion of orbital fat, the patient should be observed closely for signs of increased intra-ocular pressure. Patients who develop signs consistent with entry into the orbital cavity, e.g. ecchymosis, lid oedema or proptosis, should be monitored very closely. Intra-operative insult to the orbit should be treated immediately with mannitol 1–2 gm intravenously infused over 30–60 minutes, along with high doses of intravenous steroids; an ophtalmology consultation is obtained, and orbital massage is begun immediately. If there is impairment of vision with evidence of intra-orbital haematoma (evinced by severe pain, ecchymosis and proptosis), a lateral canthotomy or a Lynch incision with external ethmoidectomy is performed. The peri-orbita should be incised to assist drainage and decompression. Neural injury can occur if the vascular supply to the optic nerve is compromised for 60–90 minutes.

Delayed proptosis and increased orbital pressure can also occur. Post-operatively, it is important that the nursing staff be aware of possible complications and should be specifically instructed to contact the surgeon immediately in case of danger signals such as proptosis and pain in the eye.

All in all, management of lamina papyracea injury is either by abandoning the procedure (advised for beginners), or by proceeding extremely carefully (by advanced surgeons). Occasionally, the lamina itself may be dehiscent, and may pose the same problems.

Intra-orbital haemorrhage is of grave significance. On waking up, the patient complains of severe pain in the affected eye. A gradual proptosis occurs, and vision may be compromised, and the pupil reacts sluggishly. Immediate steps must be taken to reduce the intra-orbital pressure, and to decompress the optic nerve via a lateral canthotomy. If this does not succeed, an external decompression is resorted to. In addition to these measures, the patient must be given mannitol, high doses of steroids and diuretics.

Diplopia may occur due to direct or indirect injury to the medial rectus muscle or its neurovascular supply. This may be due to direct injury, cautery or laser. Diplopia may be related to oedema and is temporary; if a persistent diplopia develops, the treatment is strabismus surgery, which may not resolve the condition completely.

Subcutaneous orbital emphysema may result from the entry of air into the lamina papyracea, usually due to a Valsalva manoeuvre (vomiting, nose blowing). This is temporary, and resolves within a week.

Skull base trauma leads to a *cerebrospinal fluid (CSF) leak* just above the sphenoid ostia or sphenoidotomy openings (more commonly lateral lamella of the cribriform plate). The cribriform plate and fovea ethmoidales are other sites of injury. CSF leaks are usually detected endoscopically, and can be plugged directly with post-auricular temporalis fascia and muscle. Post-operative CSF leaks will often close spontaneously, but such patients require antibiotics and close monitoring for continuing leaks. Persistent leaks require neurosurgical assessment and a craniotomy may be needed. Sphenoid sinus breach can occur from forceps biting on the superior wall. Leakage may be controlled with packing, fibrin glue combining thrombin, calcium chloride and cryoprecipitate with a muscle plug has been used to close the leak under endoscopic guidance. An important guide in FESS is the middle turbinate, working along its lateral surface avoids injury to the cribriform plate. The base of the skull is often yellowish in colour, delineating it from the ethmoid complex. Also, in the majority of cases, the ethmoid and sphenoid anterior wall are of egg-shell consistency. When great difficulty is encountered during removal of disease or extremely hardened bone is apparent, it is prudent to withdraw and re-evaluate surgical anatomy. Patients with chronic disease will often develop thickened bone; also, those with repeated interventions may have distorted anatomy and great care has to be taken in these cases.

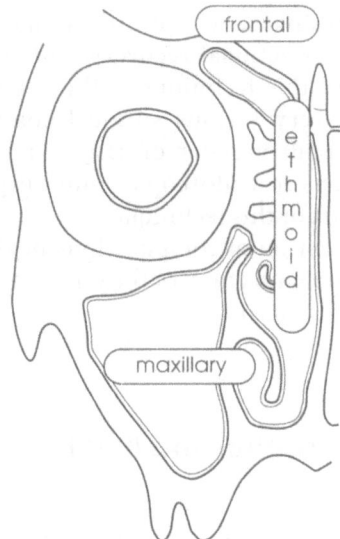

Fig. 11.9. Note the proximity of the paranasal sinuses to the orbit.

Post-operative complications include *synaechia*, without doubt the most common problem occuring with endoscopic sinus surgery. Because the middle turbinate is often preserved, its raw lateral surface apposes the lateral wall of the nose, and scarring can occur. Therefore, meticulous post-operative care is necessary. The surgeon should lyse all adhesions, which usually occur anteriorly. It should be noted that the middle turbinate has a natural tendency to move laterally, contributing to synaechia formation. If persistent adhesions block the middle meatus, a revision procedure is necessary. Finally, antrostomy closure may occur if the opening is not wide enough; lining the opening with mucosa helps in maintaining patency.

High Risk Areas in Endoscopic Sinus Surgery: Prevention of Complications

T. Ohinishi

Endoscopic sinus surgery is an excellent modality for treatment of chronic or recurrent sinusitis. It enables minimally invasive surgery for precise resection of disease within the paranasal sinuses for a better functional recovery. The only major drawback of this technique is the occurrence of potentially very serious surgical complications in a very small number of cases. Prevention of complications in endoscopic sinus surgery is an essential part of this technique.

The prevention of complications begins before the operation with study of the CT scan preferably with the radiologist.

CT Scan: Coronal and Axial

Routine examination of the CT scan of the sinuses is important as the patient may have anatomical variations in the

- paranasal sinuses
- base of the skull
- in the course of the arteries and nerves

The following anatomical sites must be carefully examined by the surgeon prior to the operation:

1. The roof of the ethmoid sinuses. The most frequent site of surgical injury is the lateral lamina of the cribriform plate as it is extremely thin and injury can lead to a CSF leak. This slanting lateral wall usually forms a gradual slope towards the roof of the ethmoid sinus.

2. The cribriform plate. In some cases the cribriform plate extends laterally into the ethmoid sinus creating a right-angled corner within the sinus. The thin bony wall in this area is often seen with a small bony defect and dehiscence. Simple stripping of the mucoperiosteum may compromise the defence system against infections. Moreover the dura mater in this area is intimately adherent to the thin bony wall and simple elevation of bone in this area may tear the dura mater creating a CSF leak.

3. The lamina papyracea. This is sometimes very thin, fragile, or dehiscent as a result of previous operation and/or longstanding multiple nasal polyps.

4. Dehiscence and unusual thinning as the patient may have had previous surgical interventions and resulting bony defects. A menin-

goencephalocele may present as a large nasal polyp through a defect in the fovea ethmoidalis or cribriform plate. The level of the anterior and posterior ethmoidal artery and its protrusion in the ethmoid sinus can be seen in the coronal view. Any difference in the height of the right and left anterior ethmoidal artery should be noted and kept in mind during operation.

In the axial CT scan the surgeon should pay particular attention to the optic nerve in relation to the posterior ethmoids where it is more likely to be damaged than the sphenoid sinus.

Haemostasis

Proper haemostasis is very important to obtain a clear operative field, thus allowing proper identification of various surgical landmarks and thereby preventing complications. Effective haemostasis should be achieved by adequate preparation of the nose and meticulous infiltration around the anterior and posterior ethmoidal arteries.

Through the microscopic observation Ohinishi (1981) has identified five main areas of the roof of the ethmoid sinus where surgical complications are likely to occur during endoscopic sinus surgery:

1. Medial wall of the ethmoid sinus or lateral lamina of the cribriform plate

2. Along the course of the anterior ethmoidal artery or nerve

3. Around the anterior origin of the middle turbinate or conchal lamina

4. Antero-lateral aspect of the roof of the ethmoid sinus

5. Area around the posterior ethmoidal artery or nerve.

Figures 11.10 to 11.14 show operating microscopic findings of the roof of the ethmoid sinus with natural dehiscence, indicating that defect or dehiscence in the roof of the ethmoid sinus is not a rare occurrence.

Complications in FESS   **85**

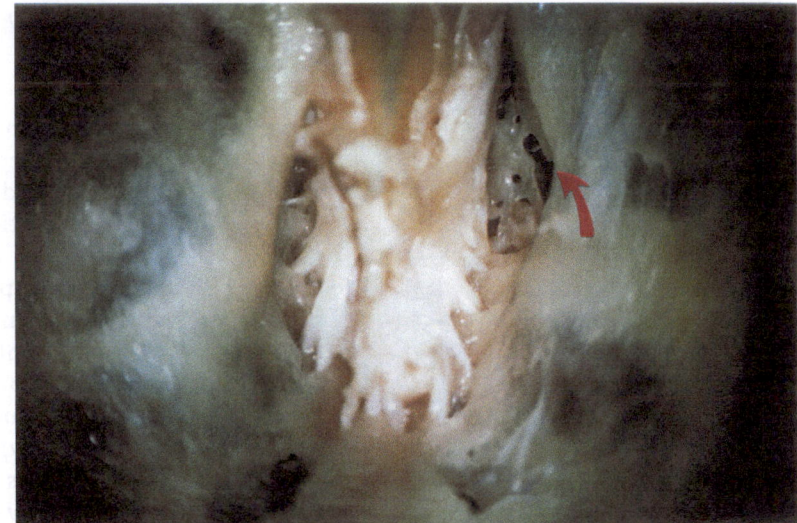

Fig. 11.10. Lamina cribrosa and the lateral wall: view from the intracranium, note multiple dehiscence in the lateral lamina of the right cribriform plate and multiple perforations for the olfactory fila. Top of the picture is anterior. Arrow shows multiple dehiscence in the lateral lamina of the right cribriform plate.

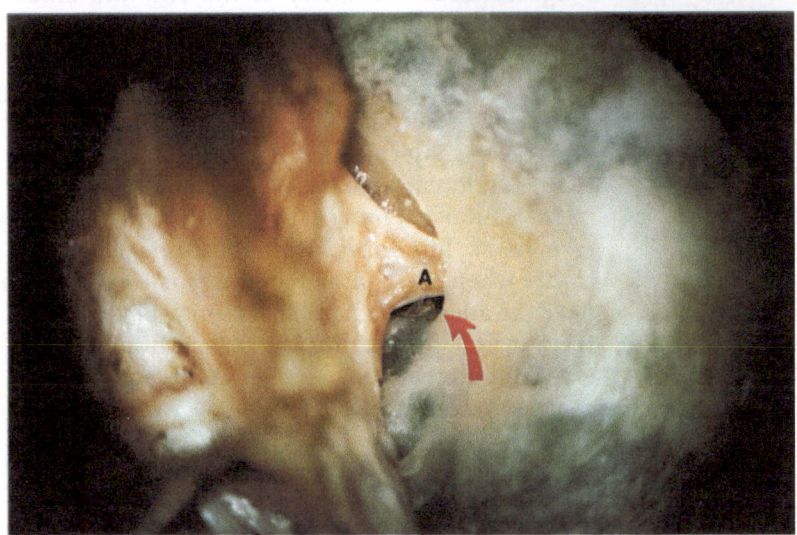

Fig. 11.11. Insertion of the right anterior ethmoidal artery (A). View from the intracranium. Note a defect of bone around the passage of the right anterior ethmoidal artery. Top of the picture is anterior. Arrow shows dehiscence around right anterior ethmoidal artery.

Fig. 11.12. Roof of the right ethmoid sinus, view from the sinus side. Note the course of the anterior ethmoidal artery (A) from the right orbit, through the lamina papyracea, to the ethmoid sinus and the defect of bone along the entire course of the anterior ethmoidal artery within the ethmoid sinus. Top of the picture is anterior. Arrow shows dehiscence along the entire course of the anterior ethmoidal artery.

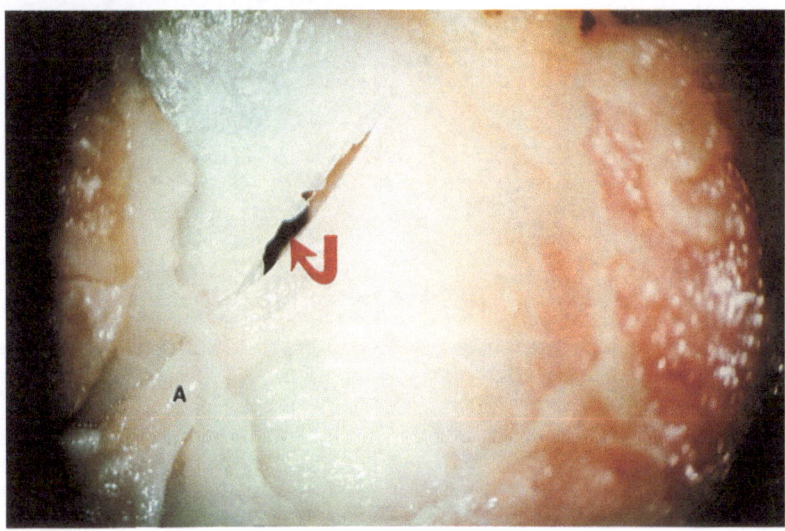

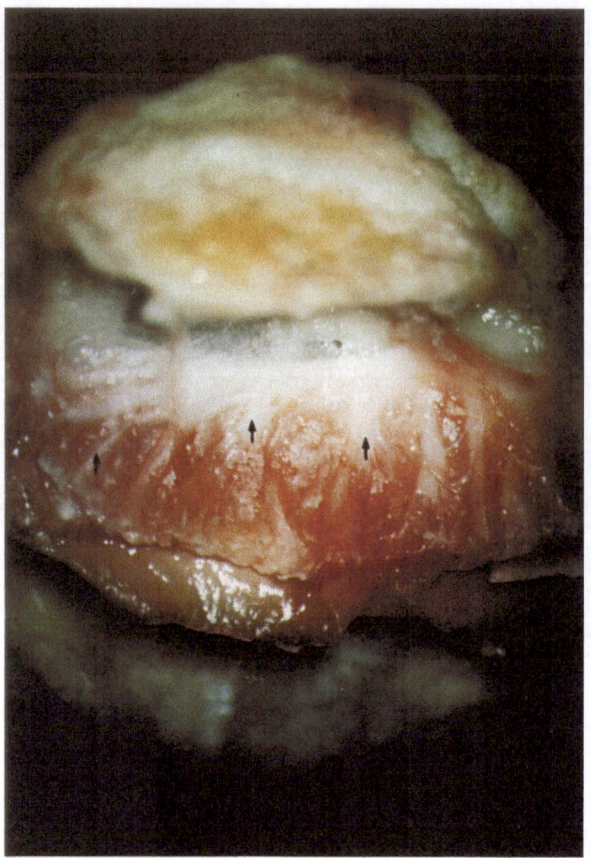

Fig. 11.13.   Upper lateral wall of the right nasal cavity, note abundant distribution of the olfactory fila (arrow) on the upper nasal turbinate and the lateral wall as seen after resection of roof of the ethmoid sinus. Right of the picture is anterior.

High-Risk Areas

Relatively high rates of serious complications have been reported by Stankeiwicz (1987, 1989), Freedman and Kern (1979) and Maniglia (1989) due to violation of the orbit and skull base. Awareness of each high risk area during sinus surgery is of paramount importance in the prevention of complications.

I have identified the following five high-risk areas that would be encountered during endoscopic sinus surgery:

Lamina papyracea. The lateral wall of the ethmoid sinus consists of lamina papyracea, the thin medial wall of the orbit, which is a convex bulge towards the cavity of the ethmoid sinus. Figure 11.15 shows an endoscopic view of the lamina when fully exposed. This is the site of relatively frequent injuries during ethmoid sinus operation. Surgical injury of the lamina papyracea may cause a simple prolapse of fatty tissue, diplopia when the medial rectus is injured, intra-orbital haemorrhage or infectious and in rare cases blindness. Complications are more severe when the lamina papyracea is traumatised near the apex as the optic nerve may be damaged. Intraorbital hematoma can cause blindness by extension to the optic nerve or compression of the central retinal artery.

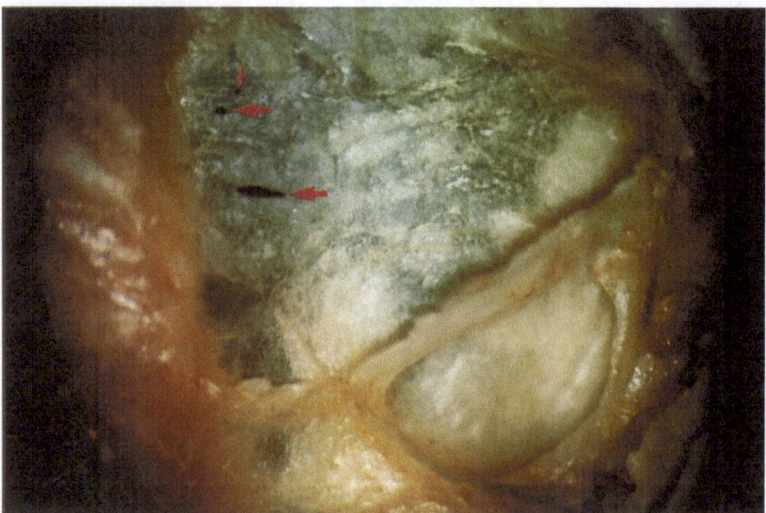

Fig. 11.14.   Roof the right ethmoid sinus after the dura mata and the mucoperiosteum have been removed. View from sinus cavity, note the thin bony roof of the right posterior ethmoid sinus and three small dehiscences (arrow).

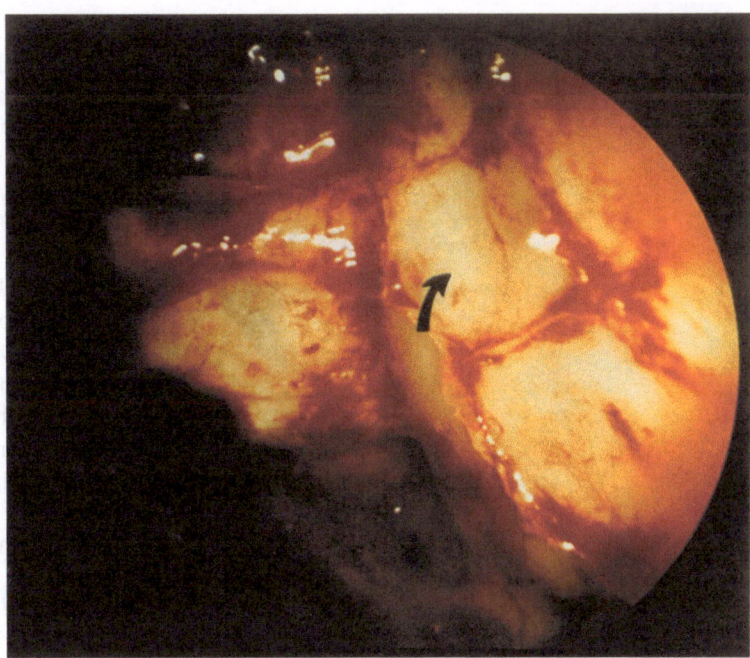

Fig. 11.15. Lamina papyracea (arrow), left ethmoid sinus.

The roof of the ethmoid sinus around the anterior ethmoidal artery. The anterior ethmoidal artery usually travels beneath the roof of the ethmoid sinus along with the nerve. There are elevations of the bony wall at the medial and lateral ends of the bony canal containing the artery. When injured it may lead to orbital haematoma in the lateral wall and CSF leakage or intracranial infections in the medial wall. Figure 11.16 shows a case where the anterior ethmoidal artery and nerve, without bony canal, course below the roof of the ethmoid sinus. This area has the unique anatomical features characterised by thin bony walls, a narrow cavity that tapers towards the ostium of the frontal sinus. Even in minor injury to this thin wall may tear the dura mater and can cause CSF leak.

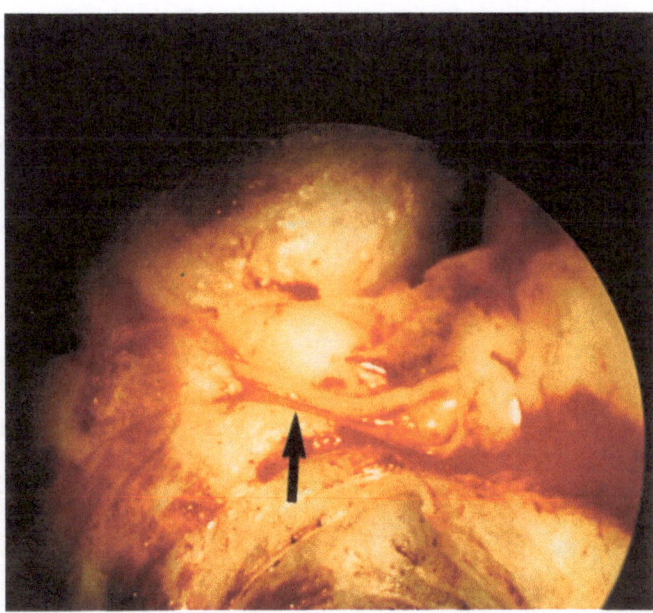

Fig. 11.16. Anterior ethmoidal artery and nerve (arrow), left ethmoid sinus.

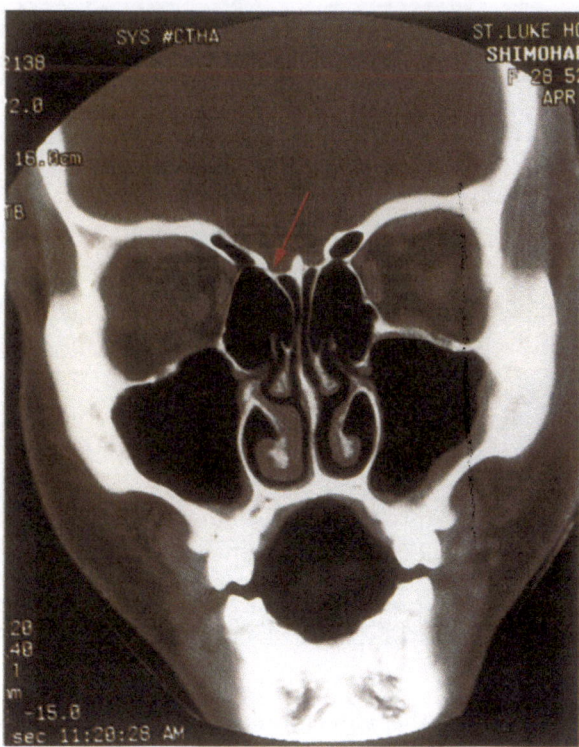

Fig. 11.17. CT findings of the lateral lamina of the cibriform plate (arrow) and the anterior ethmoidal arteries.

Lateral lamina of the cribriform plate. The medial wall of the anterior ethmoid sinus usually extends upwards above the level of the lamina cribrosa, which is the lateral wall of the olfactory bulb. This wall often bulges into the sinus cavity as is shown in the CT scan of the paranasal sinuses in Fig. 11.17. This bulging is a likely sight of surgical trauma during removal of disease in the frontal recess area. After penetrating the lamina cribrosa, the olfactory filaments distribute abundantly in the bony plates of the superior and middle tribunate which are the medial wall of the anterior ethmoid sinus. Because of these penetrations the medial wall of the anterior ethmoid sinus occasionally has bony dehiscence which may serve as a route to intra-cranial infections when damaged. Figure 11.18 shows an endoscopic view of the lateral lamina of the cribriform plate.

Ethmoid roof near posterior ethmoidal artery. The posterior ethmoidal artery travels in the roof of the posterior ethmoid sinus. The artery usually courses above the bony roof which is thicker than the roof of the anterior ethmoid sinus, and is hidden behind the bony plate. In some cases the artery, with its surrounding thin bony canal, travels beneath the bony roof. Damage to this artery may cause significant bleeding. Figure

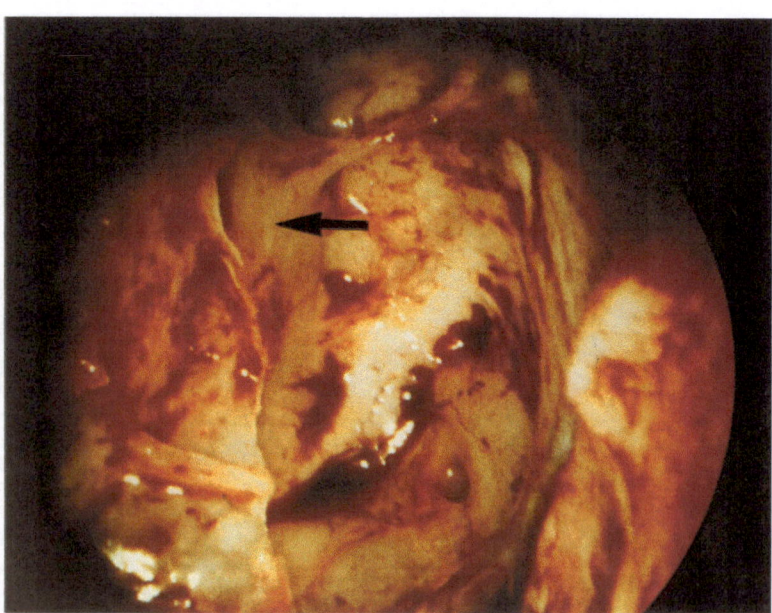

Fig. 11.18. Lateral lamina of the cribriform plate (arrow), left ethmoid sinus.

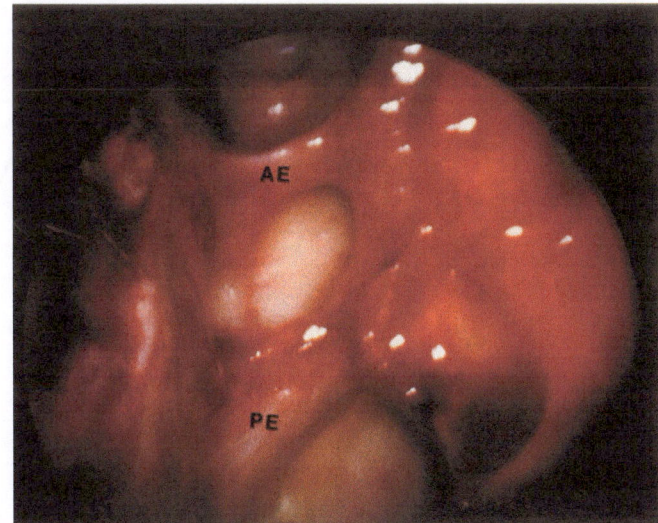

Fig. 11.19.   Posterior ethmoidal artery (PE) with the anterior ethmoidal artery (AE), right ethmoid sinus.

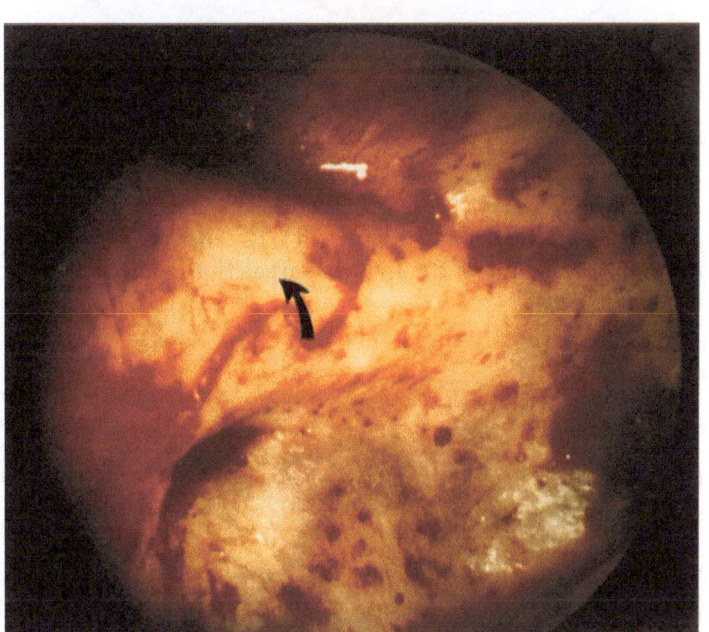

Fig. 11.20.   Optic canal (arrow) at the bordering area between the sphenoid and ethmoid sinuses, right sphenoid sinus.

11.19 shows a case where a posterior ethmoidal artery travels underneath the sinus roof, posing a risk of injury.

The bordering area between the sphenoid and posterior ethmoid sinuses. The bony bulge of the optic nerve can be seen in this area during surgery. Figure 11.20 shows such a bulging of the optic canal in the sphenoid sinus. However, injury to the nerve may occur at the area bordering the sphenoid and ethmoid sinuses where the optic canal is obscure. An attempt to remove the thick buttress between the two sinuses poses a risk of

injury to the nerve that may lie superficially to the sinus wall. The surgeon should also be aware of Onodi cells (excessive pneumatisation of the posterior ethmoidal cell) where the optic canal protrudes into the posterior ethmoid sinus. The internal carotid artery courses along the lateral surface of the sphenoid bone within the cavernous sinus causing a slight bony bulge into the sinus cavity. Injury to the artery may produce profuse and life-threatening bleeding into the sinus and the intracranial space. Craniotomy and clamping the artery may become necessary to

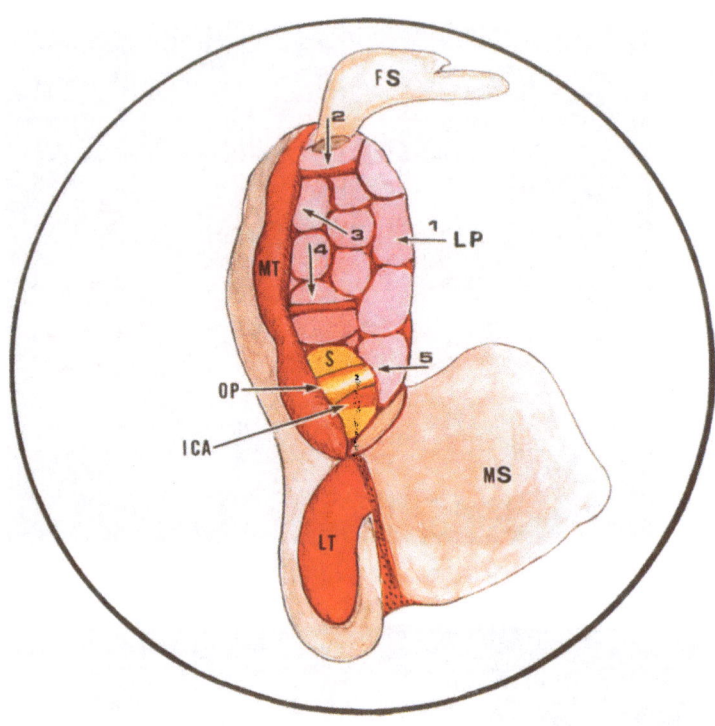

Fig. 11.21. Schematic drawing showing the high-risk areas in the left ethmoid sinuses. FS, frontal sinus; MT, middle turbinate; OP, optic nerve; ICA, internal carotid artery; S, sphenoid; IT, inferior turbinate; MS, maxillary sinus; LP(1), lamina papyracea; 2, anterior ethmoidal artery; 3–4, anterior ethmoidal cells; S, posterior ethmoidal cells.

prevent a catastrophe. Figure 11.21 shows a schematic drawing of the five-risk areas in the left ethmoid sinus.

Conclusion

The use of endoscope in sinus surgery has enabled us to visualise minute details of the structures of the paranasal sinuses and at the same time allows us to perform meticulous surgery (Ohinishi *et al.* (1990). Our previous study indicated that serious surgical complications in endoscopic sinus surgery are likely to occur when the surgeon is in haste to complete the operation owing to other commitments. As Ohnishi *et al.* (1993) indicated, a composed and calm attitude in the surgeon is an important requirement for sure and safe endoscopic sinus surgery. Perhaps most important is that the surgeon should be able to see in his or her mind the vital structures on the other side of the thin bony walls being worked upon.

Bibliography

Freedman HM, Kern EB (1979) Complications of intranasal ethmoidectomy: a review of 1000 consecutive operations. Laryngoscope 89: 421–434

Maniglia AJ (1989) Fatal and major complications secondary to nasal and sinus surgery. Laryngoscope 99: 276–283

Ohnishi T (1981) Bony defects and dehiscences of the roof of the ethmoid cells. Rhinology 19: 195–202

Ohnishi T, Esaki S, Iwasaki M; Tachibana T (1990a) Endoscopic microsurgery of the ethmoid sinus. Am J Rhinol 4: 119–127

Ohnishi T, Esaki S, Iwasaki M; Tachibaba T (1990b) Endoscopic microsurgery of the ethmoid sinus. Am J Rhinol 4: 119–127

Ohnishi T, Tachibana T, Kaneko Y, Esaki S (1993) High-risk areas in endoscopic sinus surgery and prevention of complications. Laryngoscope 103: 1181–1185

Stankiewiez JA (1987) Complications of endoscopic intranasal ethmoidectomy. Laryngoscope 97: 1270–1273

Stankiewiez JA (1989) Complications in endoscopic intranasal ethmoidectomy: an update. Laryngoscope 99: 686–690

Takahashi R (1944) Clinicoanatomical studies of the canalis orbitocranialis and canalis orbit-ethmoidalis in relation to the ethmoid cells. ORL Soc 50(3): 224–240. [English version: A collection of ear nose and throat studies. Department of Otolaryngology, The Jikei University School of Medicine, Tokyo 1971, pp 174–191

Chapter 12

Prevention of Pitfalls in FESS

The prevention of pitfalls in FESS begins not at the time of operation, but as soon as the patient presents himself to the endoscopic surgeon. Such measures can be conveniently divided into three distinct phases: pre-operative, intra-operative and post-operative.

Pre-operative Measures

There are three pre-operative measures which should be taken: History taking, nasal endoscopy and a CT scan.

As in most doctor–patient interactions, history taking is the most important aspect of patient diagnosis. A positive history of allergies, aspirin sensitivity, bleeding tendencies and recent infections must be inquired into prior to operation. Patients with specific or generalised atopy do less well following FESS, and must be warned accordingly. Also, indications for surgery in this group must be based on anatomical and/or radiological assessment of the ostio-meatal complex, and not purely on symptoms. Medical therapy must be rigorously pursued before a decision to operate is taken. Aspirin sensitivity was first described by Widal in 1922, but has been in the limelight only in recent years. It presents as part of a triad of symptoms, along with nasal polyposis and asthma. Prolonged bleeding times may also be noted. The underlying aetiology is thought to be a primary connective tissue disorder in the sensitive individual. Here again results are poorer, and no false hopes should be raised pre-operatively. Operating in a recently infected patient invites trouble, as generalised congestion and mucosal oedema cause bleeding into the narrow surgical confines, thus making the procedure difficult and hazardous.

A few salient points must be mentioned for out-patient nasal endoscopy. The 4 mm 0° and 30° endoscopes are advocated routinely. The first and second passes could be performed without anaesthetising the nose, but it is recommended that examination of the spheno-ethmoidal recess and sphenoid ostium be performed with local anaesthesia such as 4% cocaine in 1 : 1000 adrenaline.

We have had cases where the patient mentions some form of "nose operation" – endoscopy reveals an inferior meatal antrostomy, at times stenosed, or associated with residual antral disease, hence a routine examination of the inferior meatus is important. Similarly, close examination may reveal an apparent polyp to be a bifid anterior end of the middle turbinate; a medially rotated uncinate process may mimic a polyp in the middle meatus.

CT scanning should not be performed in the presence of recent rhinitis and/or sinusitis, as a false picture of mucosal oedema may be presented. Also, constant dialogue between the surgeon and radiologist is necessary, especially in regard to uncinate process position, the relation of the ethmoid roof to the nasal cavity and dehiscences of the lamina papyracea, optic nerve or internal carotid artery. So also the extent of disease should be assessed.

Intra-operative Measures

Local versus general anaesthetic and ease of access are intra-operative factors which should be considered.

Local anaesthetic is ideal, as it allows the patient to return home after a relatively safe, bloodless procedure. The patient inevitably alerts the surgeon if he approaches the lamina papyracea and/or skull base; however, the surgeon must anaesthetise the nose thoroughly, or the patient becomes unco-operative and the procedure tedious. Associated sepal deviations and/or external nasal deformities require a general anaesthetic.

The initial incision should be deep, and should follow the groove between the lateral wall of the nose and the caudal border of the uncinate process. A superficial incision will only lead to mucosal bleeding, and a proper infundibulotomy will not be achieved. The incision must extend up to the lower part of the uncinate process so as to facilitate a middle meatal antrostomy at a later stage in the operation. Similarly the upper part of the uncinate process must be removed properly, or else one would encounter difficulty in accessing frontal recess.

After the bulla has been removed, the lamina papyracea is identified and the forceps always kept parallel to its plane. Next comes the ground lamella, which should be identified and breached medially to gain access to the posterior cells. At this stage, the skull base must be identified by its thickness, and then skeletonised anteriorly by removing the remaining ethmoidal cell stumps. The ethmoid cavity has now been created; fine touches to its contours provides a well exteriorised cavity.

A middle meatal antrostomy often brings the surgeon up against the most diseased part of the nasal cavity, with polyps and discharge (in close proximity to the orbit) frequently distorting the view. Identification of the ostial site is easier when the lower part of the uncinate process has been completely excised. The level of the antrostomy is usually at the lower margin of the middle turbinate, just above the upper margin of the inferior turbinate. The upwards-cutting forceps must be directed downwards and laterally. For beginners, the combined approach (CAMMA) may be used. Caution must be exercised when advancing posteriorly, as branches of the spheno-palatine artery may be encountered. Post-operative stenosis is prevented by turning a mucosal flap over the antrostomy edge.

The fronto-nasal recess is left until last. A 70° endoscope is used to clear this area. As the ethmoidectomy has already been done at this stage, the almost unavoidable trickle of blood does not hamper the surgeon in his procedure. If oozing is excessive at any stage of the technique, the cavity may be packed with 4% cocaine-adrenaline strips, and the opposite side may be operated on.

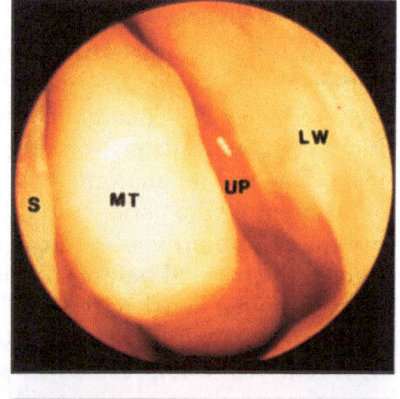

Fig. 12.1a–c. Proper nasal endoscopy often reveals abnormalities which appear different at first sight. **a** The uncinate process (UP) could well be mistaken for a polyp. **b** Closer examination shows this to be a medially rotated uncinate process. **c** Even closer examination reveals a congested and medially rotated uncinate process. S, septum; LW, lateral wall; MT, middle turbinate.

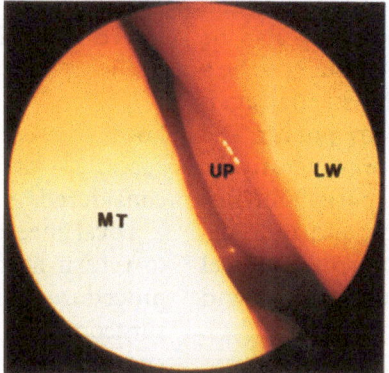

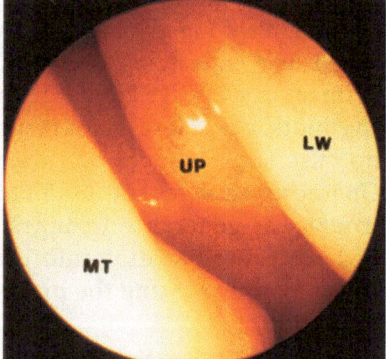

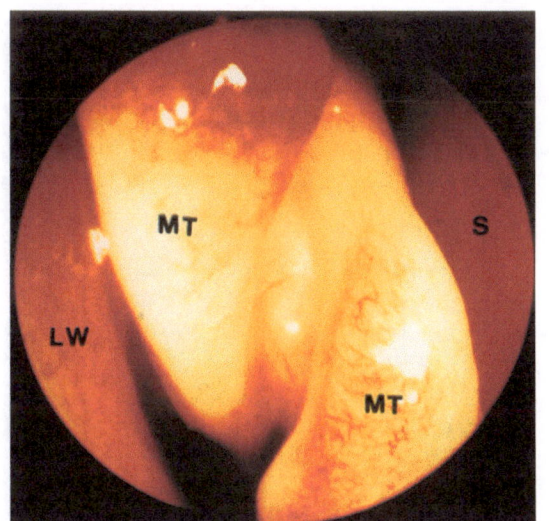

12.2

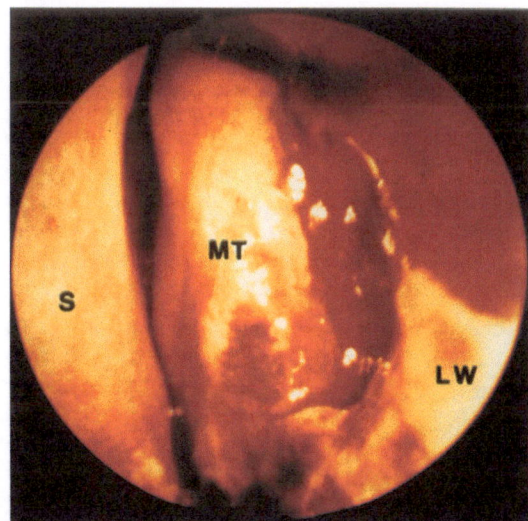

12.3

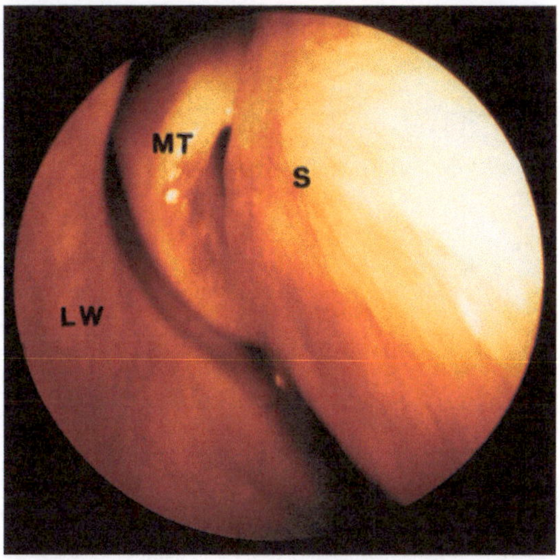

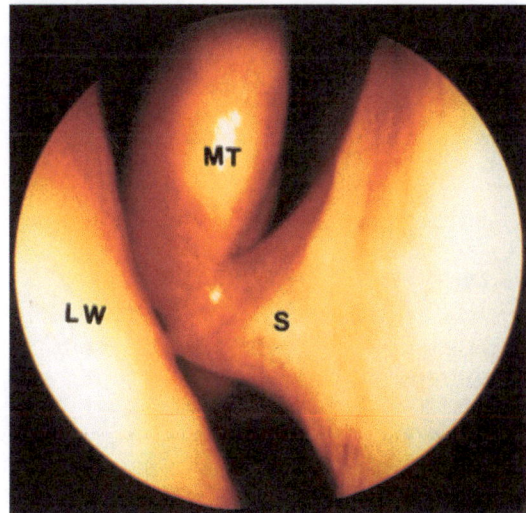

12.4

12.5

Fig. 12.2.   Similarly to Fig. 12.1, this middle turbinate shows a bifid anterior end in its longitudinal axis. Clinically, this might mimic a polyp. LW, lateral wall; MT, middle turbinate; S, septum.

Fig. 12.3.   A traumatic start causing mucosal bleeding can obscure the field, increasing the risk of complications. This should be avoided at all costs, a gentle technique is important. S, septum; MT, middle turbinate; LW, lateral wall.

Fig. 12.4.   A high deviation of the nasal septum associated with lateral rotation of the uncinate and a paradoxical turbinate is a bad combination for the novice as the operative area is very restricted. In this case, a septoplasty should be performed first. LW, lateral wall; MT, middle turbinate; S, septum.

Fig. 12.5.   A septal spur would also restrict access to the middle meatus, and trauma may lead to post-operative adhesions. LW, lateral wall; MT, middle turbinate; S, septum.

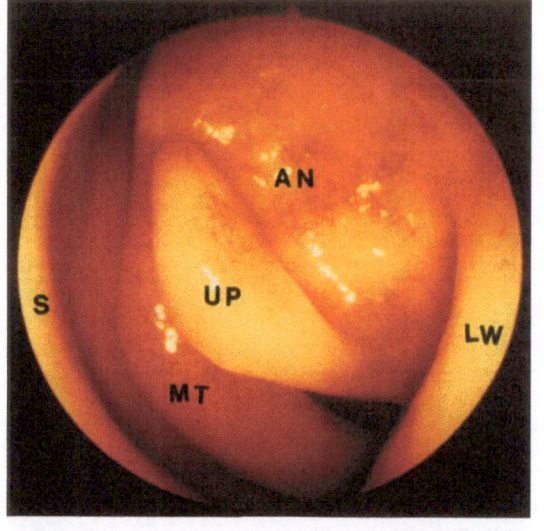

12.6

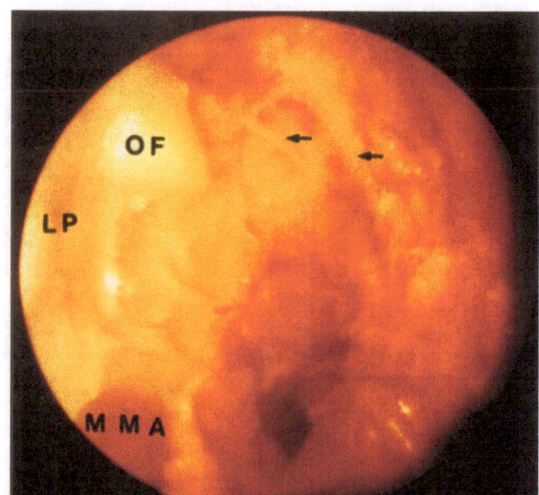

12.9

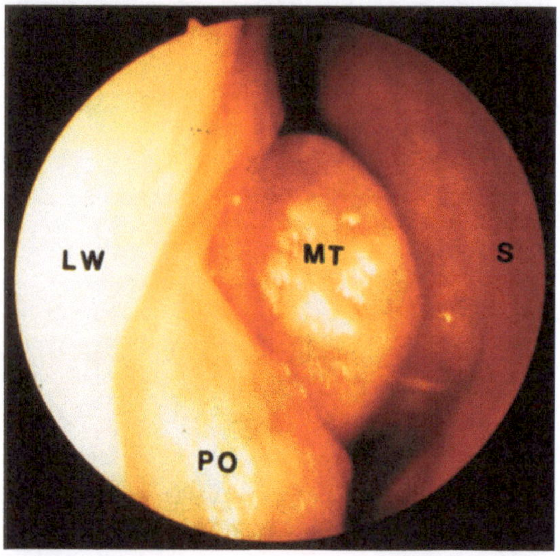

12.7

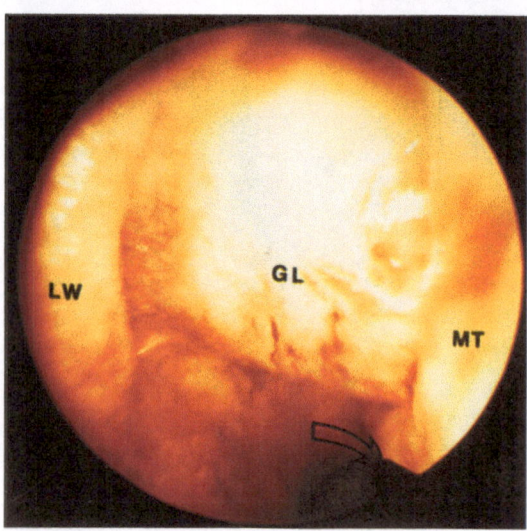

12.8

Fig. 12.6. In this case, a medially rotated uncinate process allows for easy identification of surgical landmarks, a good case for the initiate. S, septum; MT, middle turbinate; UP, uncinate process; AN, agger nasi cells; LW, lateral wall.

Fig. 12.7. In a situation where polyps (PO) protrude from the middle meatus, they should be removed gently with minimal trauma to create access to the uncinate process. LW, lateral wall; MT, middle turbinate; S, septum.

Fig. 12.8. In this case, the ground lamella (GL) is covered with thick, polypoid mucosa, and there is a danger of losing one's orientation, and of entering the posterior ethmoids unknowingly. Arrow, post-nasal space; LW, lateral wall; MT, middle turbinate.

Fig. 12.9. The skull base is identified by its nature (thick) and by small olfactory filaments running across (arrows) and the anterior ethmoidal artery in its bony canal. Orbital fat (OF) is seen as yellow in comparison with its surrounding mucosa. If pulled, it does not detach easily. LP, lamina papyracea; MMA, middle meatal antrostomy.

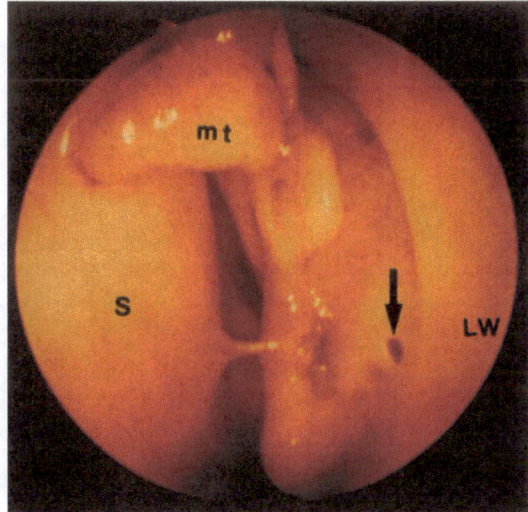

Fig. 12.10. In this revision case the normal anatomy is totally distorted due to scar tissue and incomplete excision. Such cases must not be taken lightly, and a thorough pre-operative evaluation with CT scan is required. Arrow shows the site of a probable attempt at MMA. mt, middle turbinate remnant; LW, lateral wall; S, septum.

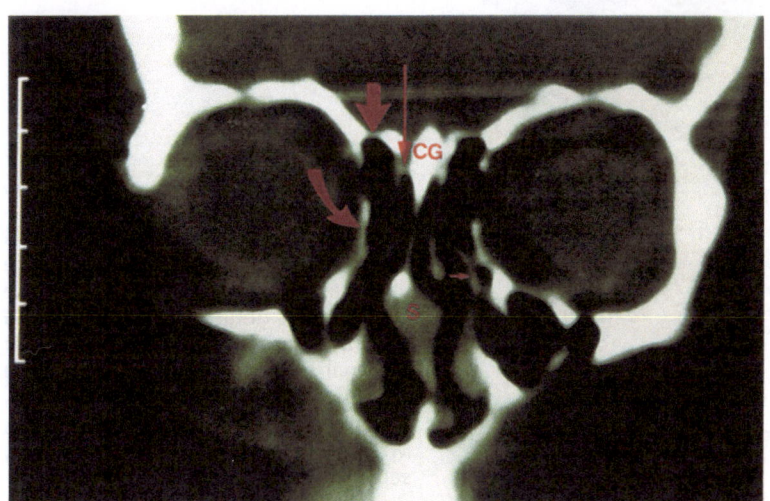

Fig. 12.11. The surgeon must know radiological anatomy of the paranasal sinuses, especially their relation to the skull base (long thin arrow). Thick arrow, fovea ethmoidales; small arrow, uncinate process; curved arrow, lamina papyracea; CG, crista gelli; S, septum.

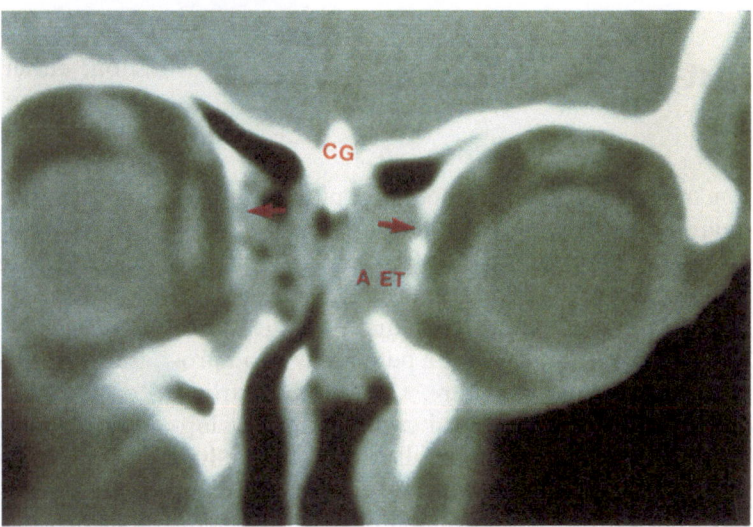

Fig. 12.12. Note the dehiscence of the lamina papyracea (arrows) due to chronic nasal polyposis and multiple operations. A ET, anterior ethmoids; CG, crista gelli.

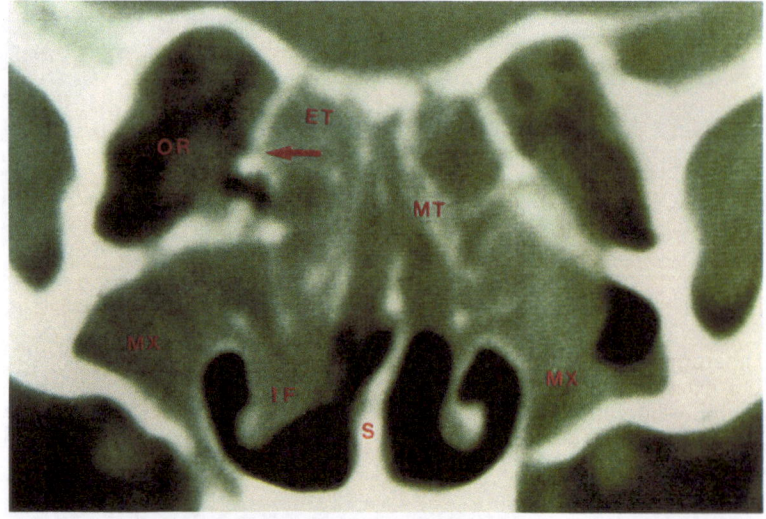

a

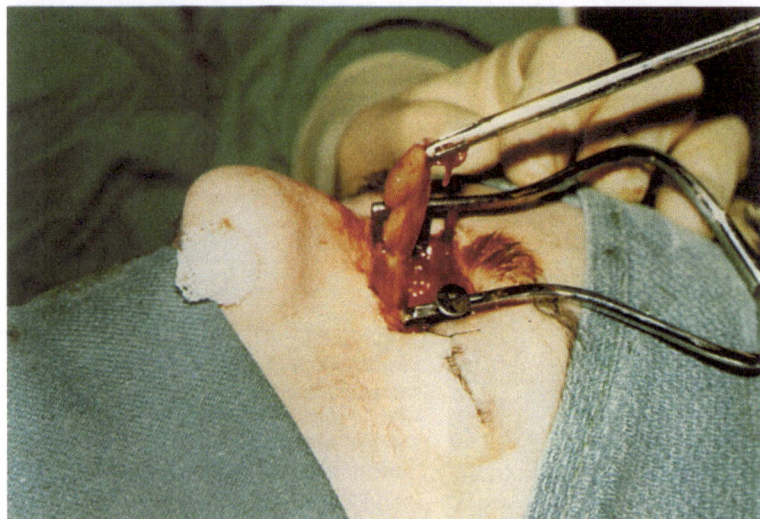

b

Fig. 12.13. a In cases of bilateral, extensive polyposis and multiple operations with distorted anatomy as seen on this coronal CT scan, FESS must be undertaken with extreme care. The arrow shows dehiscence of the lamina papyracea on the right. **b** In this case, an external ethmoidectomy may be the operation of choice. OR, orbit; MX, maxillary sinus; IF, inferior turbinate; MT, middle turbinate; ET, ethmoid; S, septum.

Post-operative Measures

The most important post-operative pitfall is inadequate after-care. In order for the newly created ethmoid cavity to heal satisfactorily, regular and frequent endoscopic toilet is absolutely mandatory. If this is not done, the surgeon may have the unfortunate experience of seeing a potentially good procedure turn into a failure. One of the earliest indicators of a mismanaged cavity is the development of adhesions. This usually occurs in the first few post-operative days. This is prevented by causing minimal tissue trauma during the operation, either with the endoscope or with instruments. The middle turbinate is gently medialised at the start of the procedure, thus preventing apposition of raw mucosal surfaces should they occur as a result of trauma. Wedge resection of the middle turbinate further modifies the ethmoid cavity, creating an anterior portal and allowing for easy access post-operatively, through which adhesions may be broken. The middle meatal antrostomy may also be compromised by the overgrowth of fibrous tissue. Furthermore, a mucosal flap should be turned inwards to line the antrostomy edges. In cases with an underlying allergy, treatment must be maintained in the post-operative period.

Chapter 13

FESS Data Analysis

Background

An analysis of our results was made possible by using a computer-compatible proforma as shown in Appendix B. Out-patient assessment, operative findings and steps and post-operative follow-up were all recorded. Symptoms were divided into the classical triad of nasal obstruction (mild, moderate, severe; right, left, bilateral), post-nasal drip and headaches and facial pains. Sequelae such as pharyngitis, laryngitis, otitis media and hyposmia were also noted. A history of asthma and aspirin intolerance were carefully recorded. Out-patient evaluation included anterior rhinoscopy, nasal endoscopy, plain radiographs and CT scans. Operative notes indicated internal architecture abnormalities and a sequential record of the procedure, while post-operative follow-up at 3 months, and then at 1, 2 or three years assessed symptoms and endoscopic findings.

This chapter presents our results in graphical fashion. It will afford the reader a clear picture of the statistics generated by our patient pool, and emphasise the need for careful and thorough documentation. We find analyses such as these act as a "rear-view mirror", telling us where we might have gone wrong, and guiding us to improvement in the future.

Over a period of 5 years, a total of 532 cases of FESS were carried out. The age range was between 7 and 87 years, with an average of 33.3 years. Just over half (51%) of patients were male. Bilateral procedures were performed in 511 patients (96%, 1022 procedures). The following results have been compiled from all patients with a minimum follow-up period of six months ($n=478$) and a maximum follow-up of 4 years.

An allergic history was elicited in 19% of cases (most of these patients were sensitive to common allergens such as house dust and pollen). Four cases of aspirin sensitivity were treated.

Secondary symptoms such as sore throats, laryngitis, middle ear effusions and smell disorders accounted for 38% of cases. A number of patients admitted to taste and smell disorders of varying degrees.

The cardinal symptoms recorded were nasal obstruction, post-nasal drip and headaches and/or facial pains. These were further graded as mild, moderate and marked. Over 60% of patients had marked symptoms.

Anterior rhinoscopy showed a deviated nasal septum in 63% of patients. These deviations, both caudal and cephalic, were often the cause of inadequate access to the ostio-meatal complex. In 76% of these, a septoplasty/rhinoplasty was carried out. Figure 13.1 summarises our anterior rhinoscopy/ nasal endoscopy or operative findings.

The following trends emerged during our study, and are worth noting

Unilaterality of Findings

Only a small number, 19 (4%) of patients had unilateral symptoms. Nasal endoscopy in these cases confirmed the presence of unilateral findings such as a conchous middle turbinate, rotation of the uncinate process, etc. These findings were further confirmed on a coronal CT scan.

Concha Bullosa

We found concha bullosae in 38% of cases, 20% of these (36 patients) showed both middle turbinates to be conchous. This figure is slightly higher than that seen in other studies, possibly due to the fact that we perform a routine wedge resection of the middle turbinate in almost all cases, hence occult conchosities are brought to light. Quite often the conchosity was in the posterior segment of the turbinate. *Almost all these patients had headaches and/or facial pains as a presenting symptom.*

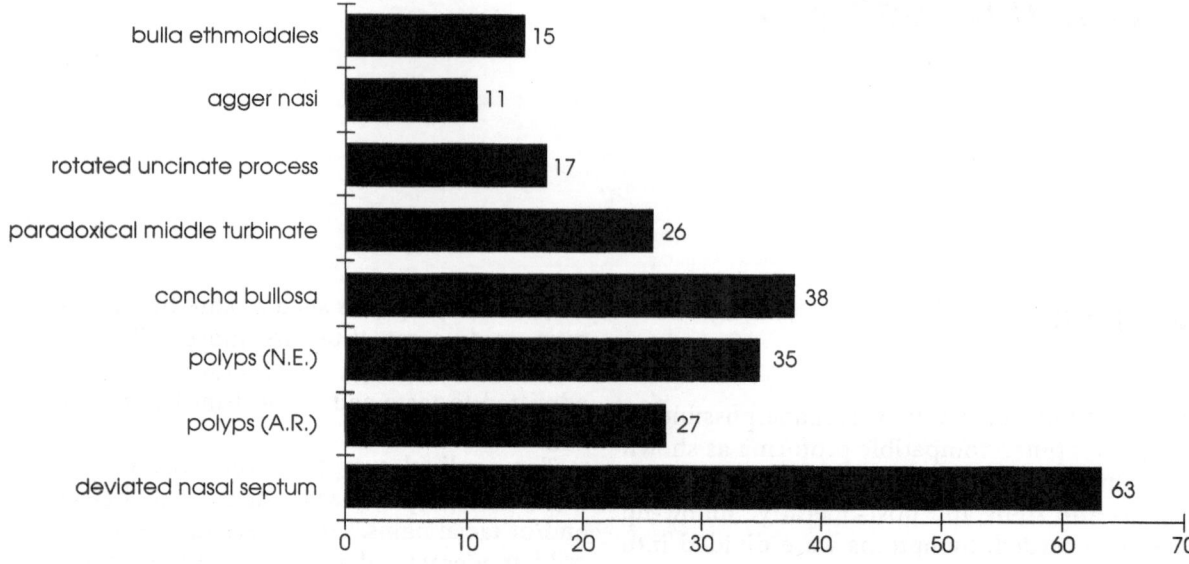

Fig. 13.1.   Anterior rhinoscopy/nasal endoscopy findings in 478 patients. Figures given are percentages; the figure for polyps (N.E) indicates findings not noted on anterior rhinoscopy.

Excising the lateral wall of the conchal sinus or wedge resection relieved the majority of these patients.

CT Findings

A small number of our patients (c. 10%) had clear CT scans in spite of being symptomatic. Once again, most of these patients suffered headaches and facial pains. Nasal endoscopy in these patients showed mild rotation of the uncinate process, muco-pus in the middle meatus, or a septal spur impinging on the middle turbinate. These findings led us to undertaking FESS in these cases.

As discussed in Chapter 6, we found plain radiograph correlation of the maxillary sinuses to have a high index of accuracy, while ethmoid assessment was poor. The key areas of the ethmoid infundibulum and the frontal recess lent themselves to assessment only by well-taken coronal CT scans. As far as comparison between CT and operative findings was concerned, we found a majority of patients with more extensive disease than that seen on film, a factor that must be kept in mind when reading the CT scan.

Post-operative Results

All FESS patients were followed up in a special Endoscopy Clinic. They were called in (initially on a twice-weekly basis, then weekly), until the cavity showed good epithelialisation, and crusting was minimal. At the clinic, they underwent rigorous nasal toilet sometimes under local anaesthesia. Their symptoms were noted on the endoscopic proforma at 3 and 6 months and then annually. The three cardinal symptoms showed the following trends over time (Fig. 13.2).

Long-term follow-up of the well-improved group (Fig. 13.3) showed nasal obstruction settled in 96.2%, headaches and facial pains in 94.4% and post-nasal drip in 92.1% (Fig. 13.4).

As can be seen in Fig. 13.4, nasal obstruction seems to be the most improved. It must be noted that obstruction may not always be due to polyps and/or septal deviations, a congestion of the nasal mucosa secondary to chronic sinusitis most often contributes too. Almost all patients who had headaches and/or facial pain had obstruction of the ostio-meatal complex. Post-nasal catarrh seems to be the most refractory symptom of the three; this may be due to the fact that hyper-

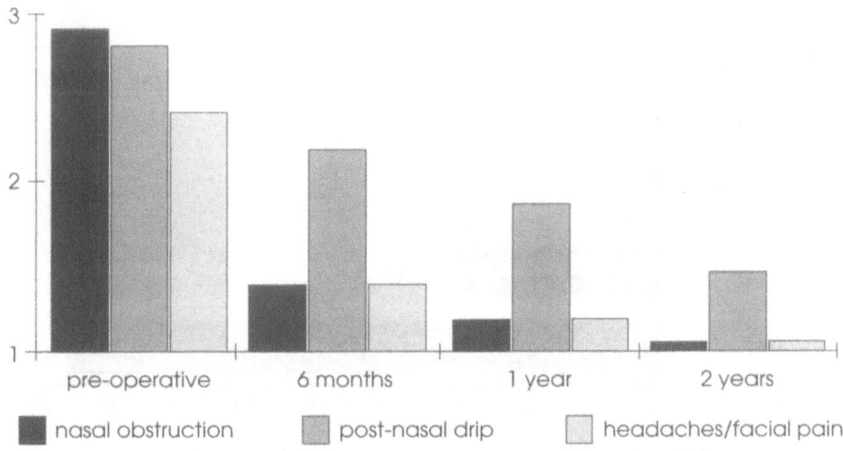

Fig. 13.2. Symptom profile in 478 patients.

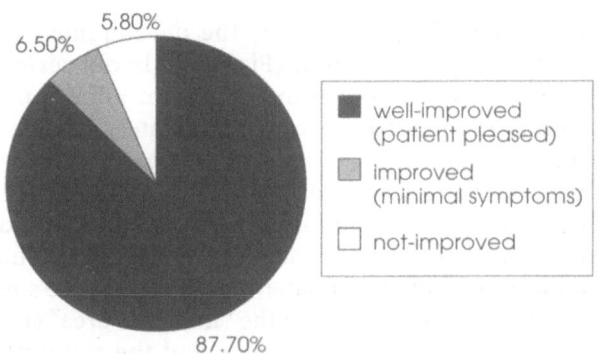

Fig. 13.3. Results of long-term follow-up of the well-improved group.

trophic sinus mucosa takes a longer time to revert back to normal; in addition, a parasympathetic overactivity might be implicated in those cases where a significant improvement was not seen.

The second group (improved – minimal symptoms, Fig. 13.3) showed a high degree of allergic symptoms, such as watering and itching of eyes, excessive, clear rhinorrhea and sneezing. These patients could have either perennial or seasonal rhinitis. The offending agent for the former group, when investigated, was most often house dust and house dust mite. The latter group showed a high incidence of sensitivity to grass pollens. Some cases of asthma or lower respira-

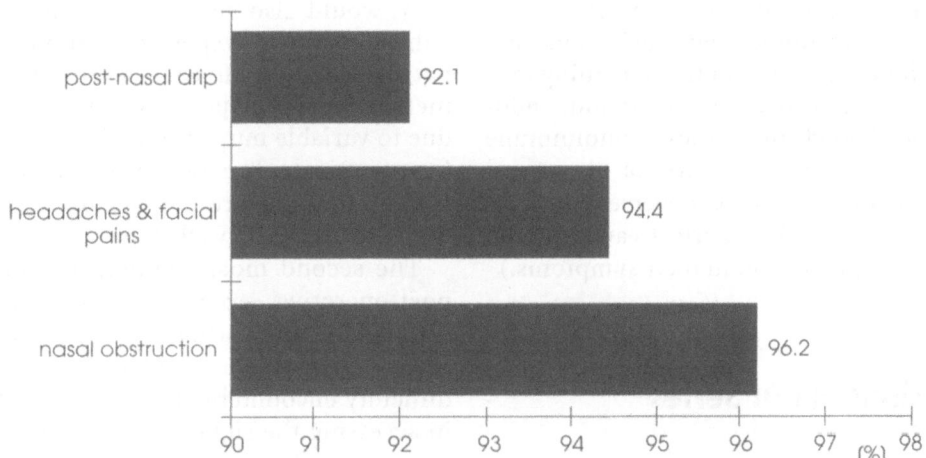

Fig. 13.4. Symptom profile in the well-improved group at 3 years ($n = 416$).

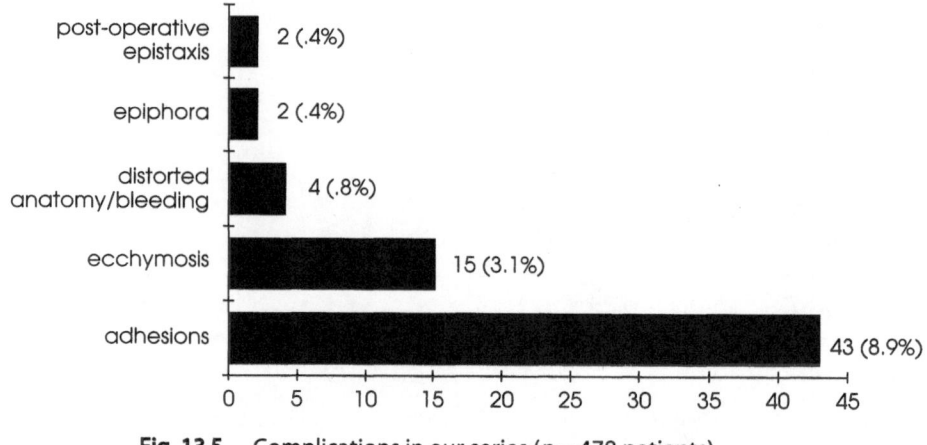

Fig. 13.5. Complications in our series (*n* = 478 patients).

tory tract infections did not therefore do as well as might have been expected.

Finally, there were a small number of patients whose symptoms remained unchanged following surgery (*n*=28, Fig. 13.3). Eleven of these had residual disease, especially in the posterior ethmoids/sphenoid. The bulk of these were in the first year; four went on to have external ethmoidectomies, while the remainder had endoscopic revision. All our cases of aspirin sensitivity (*n*=6) did badly. The classical course in these patients is an early improvement, lasting a few months at the most, followed by recurrence of disease and symptoms. One patient suffered from Kartagener's syndrome. These procedures were essentially carried out to facilitate drainage. Six cases had persistent adhesions blocking the middle meatal antrostomies and causing obstruction of the ethmoid cavities. In the remaining four patients, no obvious cause could be found; endoscopically, they had clean cavities – autoimmune mechanisms or hyper-reactivity of the nasal mucosa may play a role here. (Conversely, we have had patients with less than perfect cavities, who had near-total improvement in their symptoms.)

Complications in our Series

The most common complication both in our experience as well as in reported studies is *not* intra-operative, rather it is the development of post-operative adhesions (Fig. 13.5). In our series, 43 of 478 cases had some degree of adhesions. These ranged from some completely asymptomatic adhesions (37 cases) to those that obstructed middle meatal antrostomies and/or the ethmoid cavity, resulting in poor ventilation and drainage, requiring further surgery (6 cases). The adhesions could be unilateral or bilateral. The site of adhesions was either in the "first pass area" (i.e. between the inferior turbinate and the septum), or in the "second/third pass areas" (between the middle turbinate and the lateral wall of the nose). This must be considered against the background that 61% of our patients underwent a concomitant septoplasty or septorhinoplasty. This, naturally, would also contribute to the formation of adhesions. Our experience shows that some patients develop fibrous adhesions in spite of meticulous post-operative care. This is perhaps due to variable mucous membrane healing in different patients. The golden rule we observe is that if the adhesions are not causing any symptoms, they should be left well alone.

The second most common complication was post-operative ecchymosis (15 cases). This occurred in the earlier cases, and was predominantly right-sided. This, we feel, is due to the difficulty encountered by a right-handed surgeon in accessing the right natural os. The discolouration was only temporary, and settled in a few days. It is important to note that some of these cases had a dehiscent lamina papyracea.

Two of our cases had epiphorae, one settled after 3 weeks, and was probably due to post-operative oedema of the naso-lacrimal duct, while one did not settle after 18 months. Investigations showed scarring in the lower naso-lacrimal duct and she may need to undergo a dacryocystorhinostomy.

During the actual operation, we had significant bleeding in two cases, necessitating abandonment of the procedure, no aetiology was elicited. Two had partial procedures due to technical difficulties, one had a hypoplastic sinus. Finally, two patients bled profusely towards the end of surgery, and required post-nasal packing for 48 hours. Recovery thereafter was uneventful.

We have tried to reduce complications of adhesions by inserting a Merocel pack into the middle meatus, using splint in the ethmoid cavity, and even suturing the middle turbinate to the septum. However, our experience now shows that these measures have somewhat limited value in preventing adhesions. Only the diligent post-operative care of the ethmoid cavity has been successful in reducing adhesions significantly in recent years.

We had no serious intraorbital complications such as injury to medial rectus or optic nerve, nor any intracranial complications.

Chapter 14

Tips for Beginners

The age old chestnut, "practice makes perfect" is not, unfortunately, good advice for the initiate in FESS. Especially in today's age of medico-legal monitoring and heightened patient awareness, mistakes in this intricate region may prove very costly indeed. It must be remembered that though the surgeon tends to think in terms of statistics and series, for the patient an operation is a 100% event; it either succeeds or fails, there are usually no in-betweens. How, then, should one prepare oneself for this potentially hazardous but richly rewarding journey?

Training for FESS begins not in the operating theatre, but in the anatomy department, where an in-depth understanding of the surgical anatomy of both "hard" and "soft" parts of the nose and sinuses is gained. The next step is cadaveric dissection, and then on to the out-patient clinic, where a constant flow of patients is usually assured, and handling of endoscopes can be learnt. It is at this early stage that the initiate has to face the extremely practical problem of choice of instrument, which endoscope should he buy? As these instruments are expensive, we strongly recommend the 30° endoscope to start with, as it

serves the function of both diagnosis and operation remarkably well. If, however, this is not the case, we would then recommend beginning with a 0° 4 mm endoscope, as it allows one to develop an undistorted depth perception and orientation of the internal nasal architecture. We would suggest the 30° instrument as the next in line, and finally the 70° endoscope for advanced users.

The endoscope must be considered an integral part of the clinical examination of any patient complaining of nose and/or sinus symptoms; it is not a second-level tool to be used only in difficult cases, or in those where anterior rhinoscopy shows no clear-cut pathology. One is often astonished at the hidden pathologies that are often brought to light during endoscopic examination. The examination must be disciplined and thorough: all three passes must be undertaken irrespective of the presence or absence of pathology. Finally, the importance of careful local anaesthesia cannot be over-emphasised. Findings must be carefully documented, preferably using a clinical profile sheet, such as the one we use (see Appendix B).

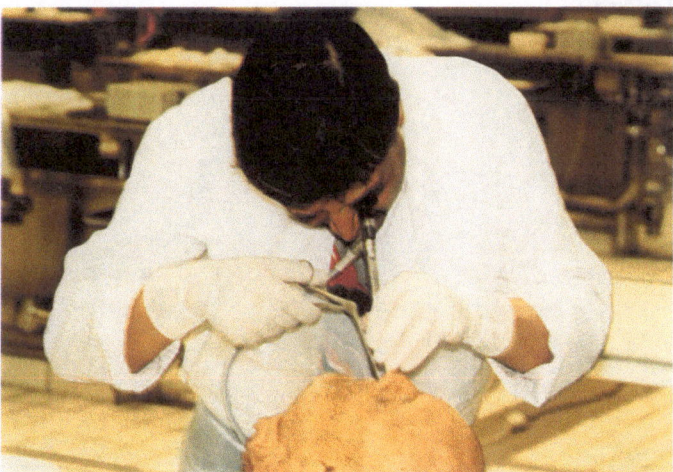

Fig. 14.1. The only way to master the technique is to dissect as many cadavers as possible.

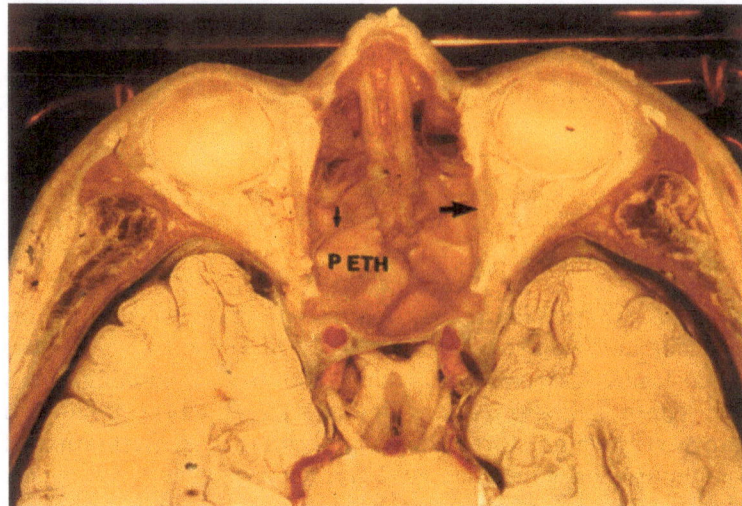

Fig. 14.2. As one advances posteriorly, one comes closer to the medial rectus, optic nerve and internal carotid artery in the posterior ethmoids and sphenoid. Also, the ethmoid cavity gets narrower; appropriate instruments should be used, and extreme care exercised. P ETH, posterior ethmoids; thick arrow, medial rectus; thin arrow, ground lamella.

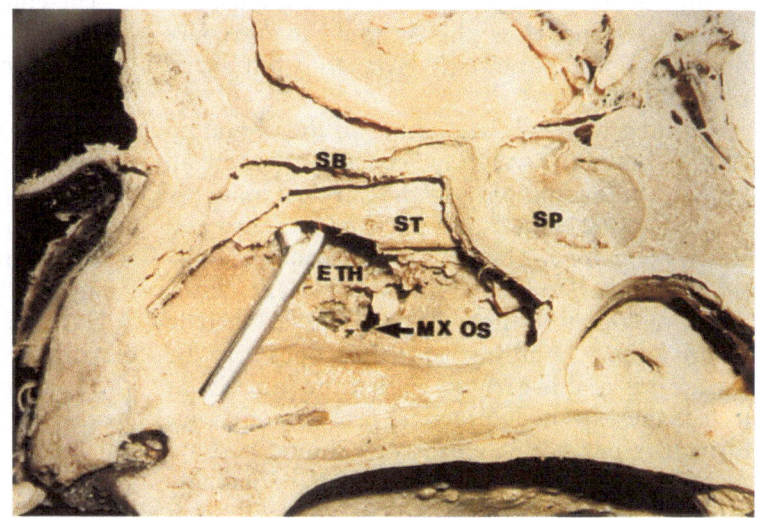

Fig. 14.3. As the instrument and the endoscope are advanced posteriorly, the dissection should follow inferiorly and medially, or else one might enter the cranium. SB, skull base; ETH, ethmoids; MX OS, maxillary ostium; ST, superior turbinate; SP, sphenoid sinus.

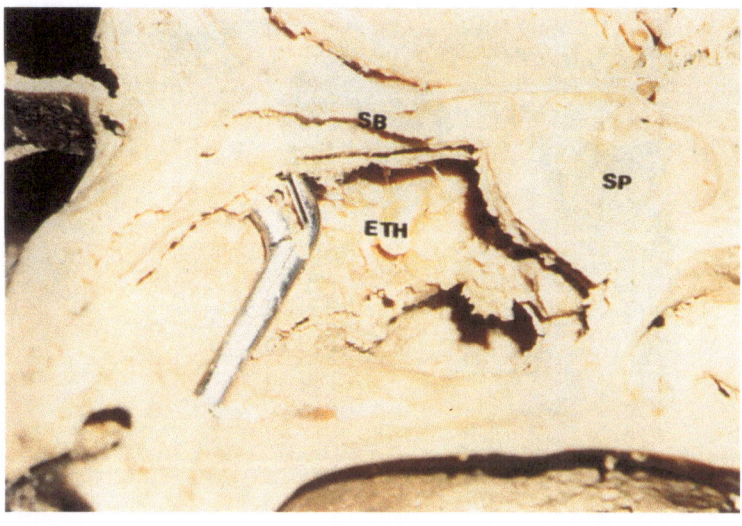

Fig. 14.4. Great care should be taken while clearing the frontal recess, any movements medially at this level will push the instrument through the thin olfactory fossa into the cranium. Hence, movements should be directed laterally. SB, skull base; ETH, ethmoids; SP, sphenoid sinus.

As the beginner acquires real-time experience of nasal endoscopy, so must he also acquaint himself with the theoretical aspects of disease in this region. This knowledge is not to be gleaned merely from textbooks, any number of hours spent in dissection and the study of the skull bones would be on too few!

The next step is perhaps the most crucial one. By now the beginner should have a clear, three-dimensional concept of the surgical anatomy of the nose and sinuses, and be comfortable with the handling of straight and angled endoscopes, he is ready for cadaveric dissection, which we consider to be absolutely mandatory, and there are no short-cuts. A useful tip at the end of the cadaveric dissection is to deliberately breach the boundaries of the cavity in order to see the relationships of the orbit and the intracranial structures. Furthermore, one of the most important skills is the ability to interpret CT scans of the nose and paranasal sinuses. Constant dialogue with the radiologist, and correlation of clinical findings with radiology reports helps to a large extent. It is often the endoscopist's job to indicate his requirements to the radiologist, who otherwise tends to give only a gross reading of his films.

Initial surgery must be confined to patients with anterior group disease, i.e. the anterior/middle ethmoids, maxillary and frontal sinuses. Revision cases or extensive disease must be avoided, as excessive scarring and distorted anatomy could pose hazards. High septal deviation patients should have their septum corrected before the actual FESS, we often perform septoplasties or rhinoplasties in order to achieve clear access to the lateral wall of the nose as a one-stage procedure.

It is advisable to begin with cases under local anaesthesia, as there is significantly less bleeding, and hence the various surgical landmarks could be easily identified. Also, the patient is aware of the procedure, and therefore warns the surgeon of pain (suggesting proximity to the orbital periosteum and skull base). The single most irritating factor for a beginner is bleeding, often caused inadvertently at the time of packing itself, or later due to coarse movements within the nose. Surgical technique overall, must be meticulous and atraumatic as in ear surgery, and frequent use of suctioning or rough movements with the endoscope or instruments should be avoided. Not only does blood obscure the field, it also stains the end of the endoscope, leading to frequent withdrawals and thereby excessive manipulation. If there is mucosal bleeding, it is prudent to pack the nose with cocaine-adrenaline strips, and wait for a few minutes. Fogging is prevented by dipping the endoscope in warm water or anti-fog solution, or by the rather ingenious method of gently touching it to the inferior turbinate. A constant watch must be kept on the eyes, as any transmitted movements could be picked up; towards this end, it is vital that the eyes remain uncovered all the time. The patient's CT scans must always be on hand, so that they can be used as a "road-map" during the operation.

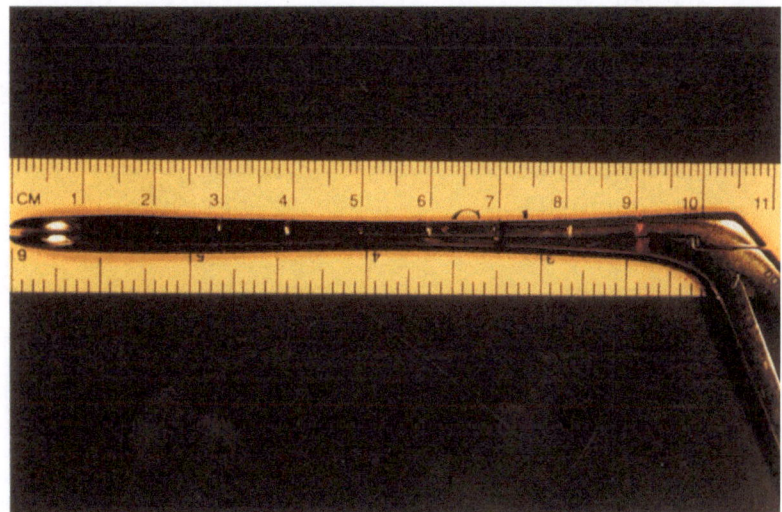

Fig. 14.5. Always be aware of the depth of the instrument within the nasal cavity from the anterior nasal spine. At 7 cm is the anterior wall of the sphenoid, and at 9 cm one is within the sphenoid sinus. Marking the forceps shaft is a useful trick.

As the learning curve is traversed, posterior sinus involvement is tackled more frequently, and cases may be operated on under a general anaesthetic. Only when the surgeon is at an advanced stage of expertise should recurrent or revision cases or extensive disease be taken on, gradually undertaking new horizons in endoscopic sinus surgery.

Ten commandments in endoscopic sinus surgery

- acquire an intimate knowledge of the surgical anatomy of the nose and sinuses, especially of the ostio-meatal complex
- evaluate patients thoroughly with nasal endoscopy and CT scan pre-operatively
- develop good endoscopic diagnostic skills using the 0° endoscope and acquire familiarity with the instruments
- perform several cadavaric dissections in order to master the technique
- remember, local anaesthesia permits a better field and is also safer. The patient simply would not allow the surgeon to enter the orbit or skull base
- avoid unnecessary trauma to the nasal mucosa to minimise bleeding
- use the CAMMA technique in the initial stages to gain better visualisation of the operative area
- do not select cases with extensive disease or a history of multiple interventions in the past
- when in doubt due to distorted anatomy, choose an external approach
- meticulous post-operative care is essential for preventing adhesions

Chapter 15

Broadening the Horizons

As the endoscope comes into wider use, its applications extend to include –

- posterior epistaxis
- mucoceles
- acute sinusitis not responding to medical treatment
- orbital cellulitis and abscess
- dacryocystorhinostomy
- inverted papilloma
- CSF leak
- frontal sinus osteomas
- orbital decompression for Graves disease
- optic nerve decompression
- pituitary tumors
- foreign bodies: nose and sinuses
- olfactory disorders: hyposmia, dysosmia
- endoscopic management of choanal atresia
- endoscopic vidian neurectomy
- endoscopic management of intranasal and eustachian tube adenoids

Endoscopic Approach to Posterior Epistaxis

The role of nasal endoscopy in the evaluation of chronic sinus disease in now universally accepted in patients complaining of nasal and/or sinus symptoms (Kaluskar 1992). As one develops the expertise in handling the multiangled endoscopes and becomes familiar with the normal and abnormal anatomy of the nasal cavity, the use of nasal endoscopy can be further extended to embrace a common clinical emergency, epistaxis, with most gratifying results. Epistaxis affects about 10% of the population showing significant episodes (Weiss 1972; Shaheen 1975). Rarely it can be fatal. (Hara 1962)

Successful management of epistaxis is directly related to the location of the bleeding point. The more common anterior epistaxis is the least dangerous as it is easily located and cauterised. On the other hand posterior epistaxis may be quite severe, and more difficult to identify and control. It usually occurs in the elderly, who are intolerant to haemodynamic change and are often associated with hypertension, arteriosclerosis and various coagulopathies. The conventional treatment calls for a nasal packing, both anterior and posterior, antibiotics and a prolonged hospitalisation with increased morbidity. This results in significant pain in the nose and swallowing difficulties due to postnasal packing.

In recent years, one of the most valuable applications of the nasal endoscope has been its use in dealing with posterior epistaxis. This has shown excellent efficacy approaching 90% (Wurman 1992), a minimal complication rate (McGarry et al. 1991) and higher degree of patient satisfaction (O'Leary and Stickney 1992).

Posterior epistaxis occurs in an inaccessible area of the nasal cavity. The main pathological change in the arteries in the nasal cavity is increased fibrous tissue in the muscularis layer of the arterial wall (Shaheen 1975) and it may be that the rigid skeleton of the arterial wall prevents its contraction. Our experience in nasal endoscopy for posterior epistaxis has revealed the source of bleeding point as follows:

- the posterior part of the lateral wall near the sphenopalatine foramen
- from the posterior end of the inferior turbinate
- the middle turbinate and its medial surface
- from the floor beneath the inferior turbinate
- the middle and posterior part of the septum

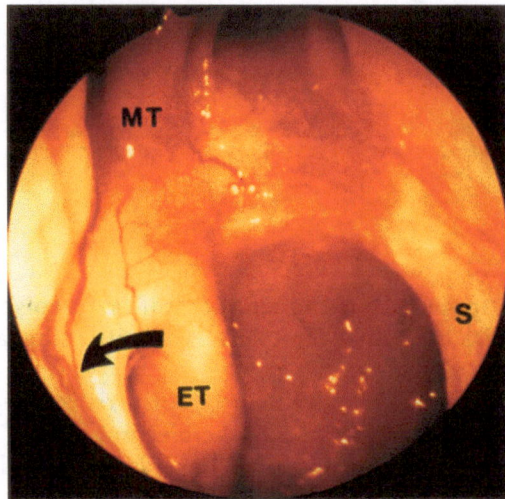

Fig. 15.1. Endoscopic view of Woodruff's plexus (arrow). ET, eustachian tube; S, septum; MT, posterior end of the middle turbinate.

- from the post-nasal space especially from Woodruff's plexus (Fig. 15.1) (Woodruff 1949).

In our experience bleeding from the Woodruff's plexus is usually a small trickle compared with the severe epistaxis from one of the branches of the sphenopalatine artery or anterior ethmoidal artery. The source of bleeding in posterior epistaxis has almost always been a single spurting blood vessel rather than engorged multiple blood vessels seen in anterior epistaxis.

Treatment Modalities of Posterior Epistaxis

Traditionally methods of treatment of posterior epistaxis are:

- anterior and posterior nasal packing with bismuth iodine paraffin paste (BIPP)
- various balloon catheters
- arterial ligation
    internal maxillary artery
    anterior and posterior ethmoidal arteries
    external carotid artery
- arterial embolisation

In practice most surgeons resort to anterior and posterior nasal packing usually performed under general anaesthesia. In intractable cases anterior ethmoidal or external carotid ligation is performed depending upon the perceived source of bleeding. The drawbacks of the antero-posterior packing are as follows:

- prolonged admission, greater than 5 days on average
- High complication rate of 68% in these patients as shown by Wang et al. 1981 and Fairbanks 1986. There is certainly an increased morbidity in the post-operative period with significant pain and discomfort. Jensen et al. (1991) have shown the complications following anterior and posterior nasal packing such as sinusitis, otitis media, aspiration, toxic shock, hypoxia/hypercapnia, myocardial infarction, cardiovascular accidents, alar and columellar necrosis and scarring, development of septal perforations and adhesions.

The alternative method of posterior endoscopic cauterisation in the case of epistaxis affords the following advantages:

- its efficacy is in the region of 90%
- it does not require nasal packing
- it can be carried out under local anaesthesia in an out-patient clinic and has an excellent patient tolerance
- most patients are treated as out-patients
- even if admission becomes necessary, the mean in-patient stay is significantly reduced
- long-term side-effects of nasal packing are abolished
- it affords an early screening method for more extensive surgery as the potential severity of bleeding is obvious.

The side-effects of posterior endoscopic cautery are few. Wurman (1988) reported transient palatal anaesthesia and considered the theoretical risk of damaging the eustachian tube orifice with scar tissue in overenthusiastic cautery. However, these are avoidable complications.

We have now successfully treated 18 patients with posterior epistaxis including one case of haemangioma on the posterior part of the inferior turbinate (Fig. 15.2). Only five patients needed hospital admission, three for overnight observation due to social circumstances and two needed 3 days admission as they were post-operative (FESS) posterior epistaxis. All others, (13 patients) were treated as out-patients following endoscopic electric cauterisation under local anaesthesia.

Posterior endoscopic cauterisation of the source of bleeding is, initially, a cumbersome procedure as the endoscope and suction or cautery equipment has to be introduced into the nasal cavity. However, this can be overcome as one gains experience in handling the endoscopes. Nasal anatomy may make the passage of endoscopes a little difficult and an occasional septal correction may be required. In cases of septal deflections, we have used 2.7-mm endoscopes for successful posterior epistaxis cauterisation without the need for septal surgery.

15.2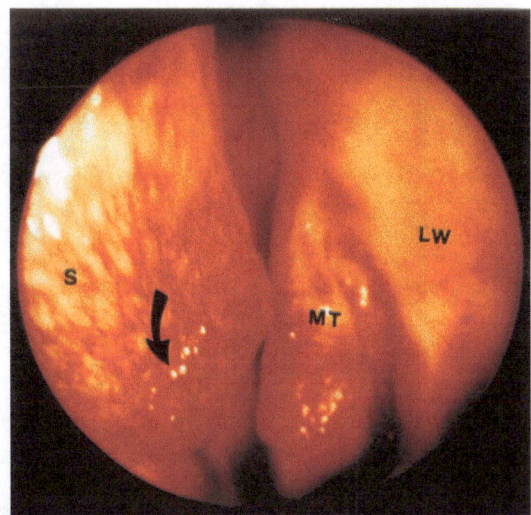

15.3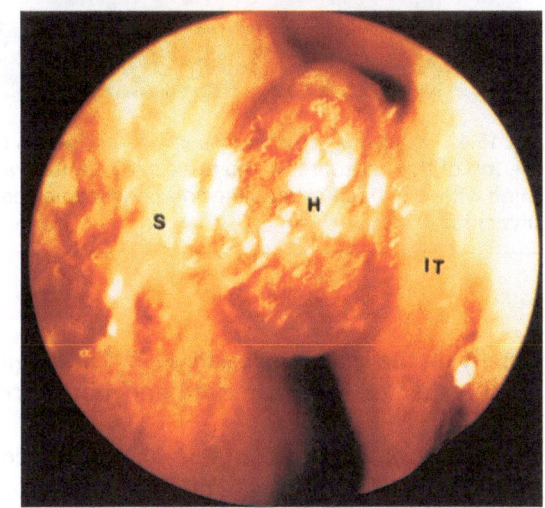

Fig. 15.2. An elderly patient was admitted with profuse posterior epistaxis. Thorough cocainisation of the nose and careful nasal endoscopy revealed a bleeding point far back on the nasal septum. This was cauterised with suction/cautery under local anaesthetic, thus avoiding a post-nasal pack. S, septum; MT, middle turbinate; LW, lateral wall; arrow, engorged blood vessels.

Fig. 15.3. A haemangioma on the posterior end of the left inferior turbinate. Multiple attempts at anterior nasal packing proved unsuccessful; however, nasal endoscopy identified the cause. S, septum; H, haemangioma; IT, inferior turbinate.

The equipment (see Fig. 15.4) used for posterior nasal endoscopy is quite common; for example:

- 4 mm and sometimes 2.7 mm 0° endoscope
- suction equipment, preferably with diathermy
- standard electric cautery equipment
- silver nitrate sticks in case of continuous oozing, e.g. Woodruff's plexus

Technique of Endoscopic Cauterisation

The patient is placed in a semi-sitting position and is given a bowl to clear blood clots into from the back of the throat. Initially 4% cocaine with 1 : 1000 adrenaline is applied on the soft Unicergel or cotton wool pledges to the nasal cavity which is actively bleeding. Usually, after a few repeated insertion of cocaine adrenaline the nose is well anaesthetised but, if necessary, anaesthesia could be supplemented by a sphenopalatine block with 1% lignocaine and 1 : 200 000 adrenaline injected at the posterior end of the middle turbinate. Sometimes a local injection of lignocaine can be made on the septum at the site of the bleeding point. A meticulous examination of the nasal cavity including various meati should be made and any blood clots removed. A bleeding point is usually seen in the form of markedly engorged blood vessels on turbinates, a large single vessel on the lateral wall, or a nipple-like projection

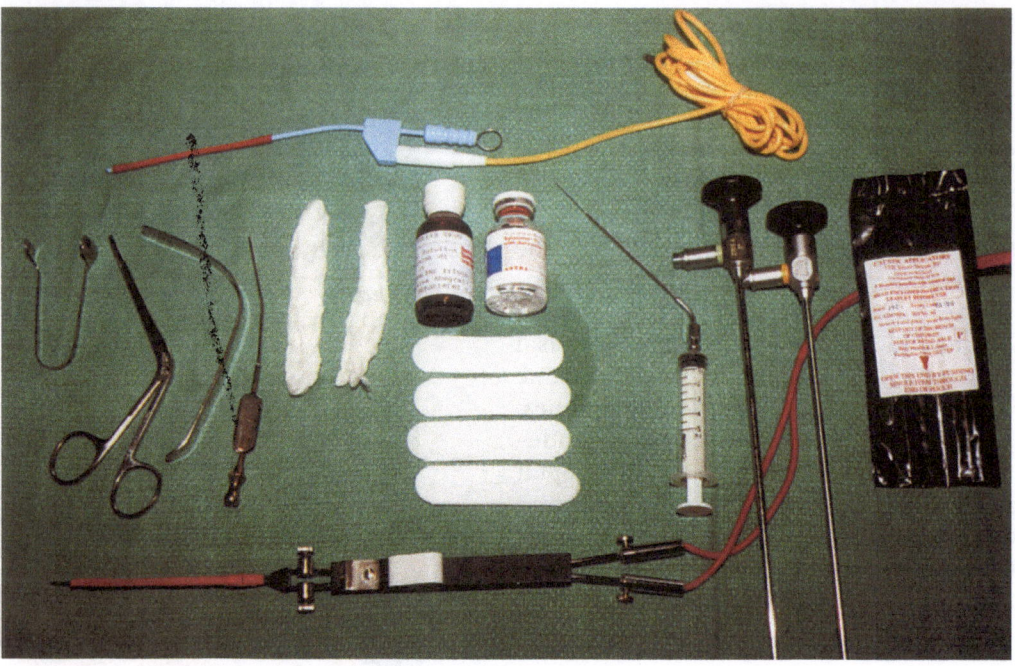

Fig. 15.4. Equipment for endoscopic cauterisation of posterior epistaxis. Note the suction cautery with insulation at the top of the photograph and the electric cautery at the bottom; 4% cocaine with 1: 1000 adrenaline and 1% lignocaine with 1: 200 000 adrenaline and endoscopic needle in the middle; far right are 4-mm 0° and 30° endoscopes and silver nitrate sticks.

usually on the septum is easily seen. The bleeding point is then electro-cauterised under endoscopic control.

We strongly recommend that nasal endoscopes should be routinely used in preference to the blind insertion of nasal packing or balloons. The morbidity and mortality associated with this most common ENT emergency can be greatly reduced. A thorough nasal endoscopy after topical anaesthesia, location of bleeding point and cauterisation should be the first-line treatment in all cases of posterior epistaxis. Nasal endoscopy in cases of posterior epistaxis is a significant major advancement for precise location of a bleeding point.

Mucoceles of the Paranasal Sinuses

A mucocele arises from the retention and accumulation of thick, mucoid secretions within a paranasal sinus, giving rise to expansion, thinning or lysis of one or more walls of the sinus. When mucoceles are infected, they form mucopyoceles. Mucoceles are lined by the epithelium. Sometimes they are misdiagnosed due to alarming neurological symptoms and signs. They need proper radiological investigation and once diagnosed the treatment is usually of marsupialisation and an adequate drainage. Approximately 65% of mucoceles occur in frontal sinuses, 30% in anterior ethmoids, (Howarth 1921; Rogers 1976). Sphenoidal and posterior ethmoidal mucoceles are rare. Maxillary involvement occurs in about 5% to 10% of cases. (Zizmor, 1974).

In his biography of Francis I, Francis Hackett (1934) recounts an illness from which the French King suffered while a prisoner in Spain in 1524. The illness described accurately follows the clinical course that an infected mucocele can take when untreated. The first documented case was reported by Dezeimerisn in 1725. However, Langenbeck in 1818 wrote the detailed description of a frontal sinus mucocele calling it a Hydatid. It was a French pathologist, Berthon in

1880, who reported the first treatment of a frontal mucocele. Onodi in 1901 described the histological characteristics of these lesions. In 1909 Rollet suggested the term mucocele. Herrnheiser presented the first detailed description of the radiological appearances of these lesions in 1926.

Aetiology

The aetiology of the mucocele is primarily that of obstruction and inflammation of the sinus due mainly to the following factors in a majority of patients:

- chronic sinusitis
- nasal polyps
- trauma either accidental or operative
- neoplasms

In a small number of patients the nature of obstruction is not clear. In these cases it may relate to anatomic variations and absence of alternative pathways. Histological examination of the mucocele confirms the chronic inflammatory process where osteolysis, new bone formation and sclerosis has been identified.

Clinical Features

Mucoceles are slow-growing lesions and hence do not cause symptoms and signs until there is involvement of the surrounding structures. Symptoms vary in general and clinical features depends upon the size, location and presence of secondary infection. The following are the common symptoms in case of fronto-ethmoid mucoceles. Slowly growing, painless, fluctuant swelling in the forehead or fronto-nasal region of the orbit just above the inner canthus. This may ultimately cause upper eye lid ptosis and proptosis with inferolateral displacement of the eye (Figs. 15.5, 15.6). Headaches, pain in the region of the swelling, diplopia, blurring of the vision and epiphora may occur. Progressive compression of the orbital contents may lead to visual impairment and even optic atrophy. Endoscopic examination may reveal bulging in the region of the middle meatus. CT scan both coronal and axial (Figs. 15.7–15.9) usually clinches the diagnosis by showing radio opacity, bony destruction, marginal bone sclero-

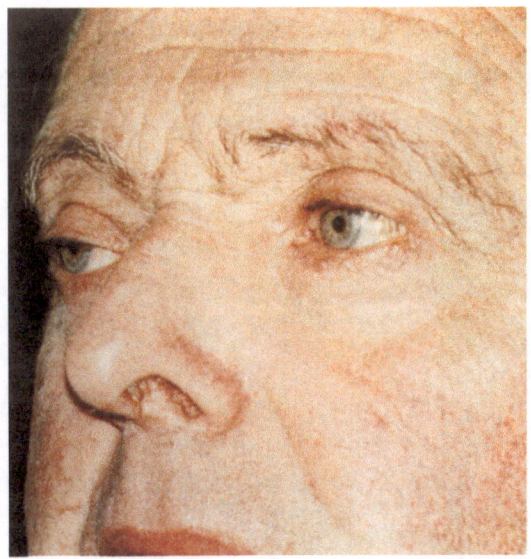

Fig. 15.5. Right large fronto-ethmoid mucocele in a 60-year-old man. Note the right proptosis. The patient had had several sinus operations in the past.

sis and loss of scalloping in case of frontal sinus mucocele. Thorough CT assessment is essential to decide a surgical approach. MRI would be useful to differentiate mucocele from neoplasms and meningoceles.

Sphenoid sinus mucoceles are uncommon and usually present with headache and opthalmological symptoms. The headaches are localised to the vertex, forehead or around the eye. Inflammation or oedema of the optic canal is usually responsible for the visual disturbances rather than direct compression.

Treatment

Prior to the advent of endoscopic surgery, patients were treated by external approach either by the Lynch–Howarth or osteoplastic procedures requiring several days in the hospital. Both these approaches have been associated with high degree of recurrence. A non-invasive endoscopic approach is much preferable in suitable cases where the mucoceles can be widely marsupialised under direct vision, avoiding external incisions and post-operative morbidity. In more laterally placed mucoceles a combined approach may be necessary.

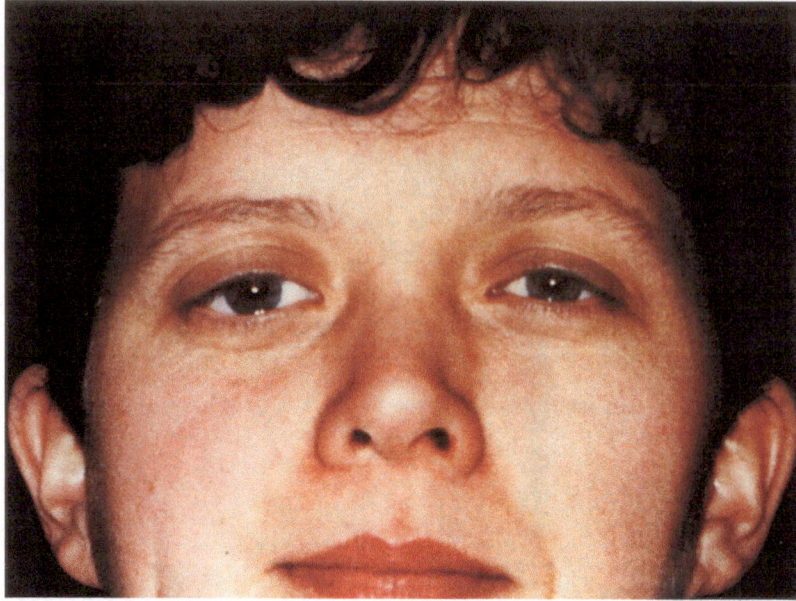

Fig. 15.6. A 32-year-old woman complaining of right epiphora and swelling of the right eye. A diagnosis of fronto-ethmoid mucocele was made which was marsupialised through the endoscope.

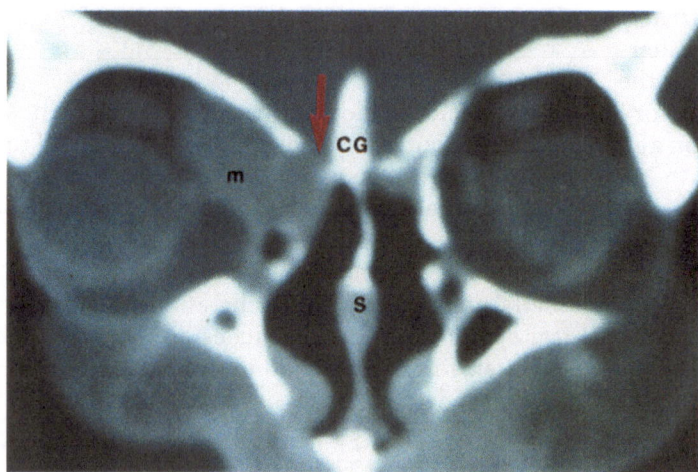

Fig. 15.7. Coronal CT scan of the sinuses. The arrow shows destruction of the bone due to mucocele. Also note the complete absence of both middle turbinates. M, fronto-ethmoid mucocele; CG, crista galli; S, septum.

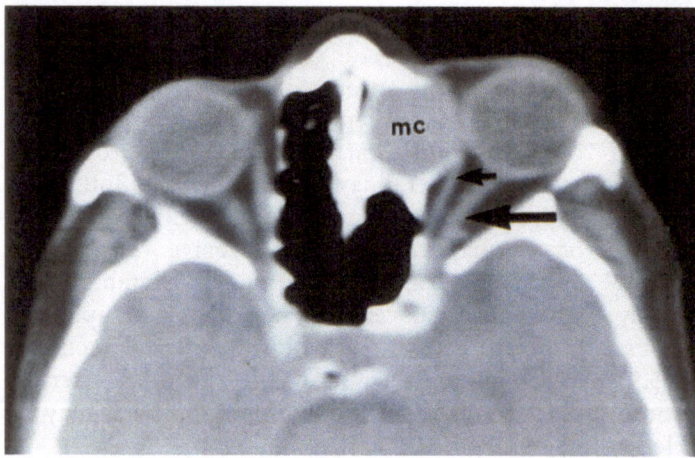

Fig. 15.8. Axial CT scan showing mucocele of the ethmoid sinus causing minimal unilateral proptosis (mc); medial rectus (short arrow); optic nerve (long arrow).

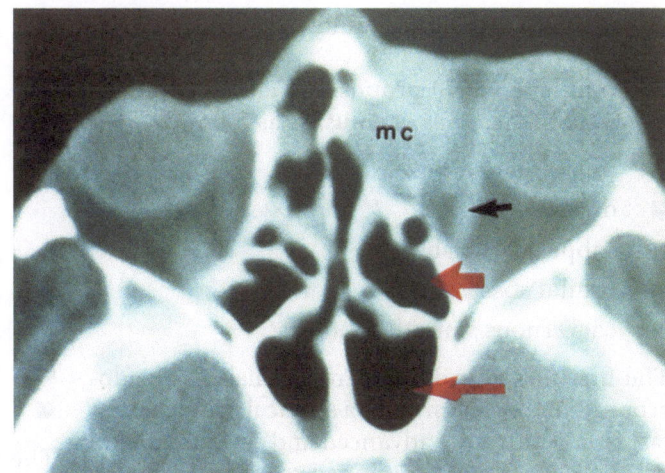

Fig. 15.9. Axial CT scan showing mucocele of the fronto-ethmoid sinus causing unilateral proptosis (mc); medial rectus muscle (small arrow); posterior ethmoid sinus (short arrow); sphenoid sinus (long arrow).

The operation is performed either under local or general anaesthesia as a day-case procedure. After topical decongestion of the nasal cavity a 4-mm, 0° endoscope is used and after identifying surgical landmarks the inferior expansion of the mucocele is uncapped with a sickle knife. The opening of the mucocele is then widely enlarged with an upward-cutting forceps and the turbid inspissated mucus is removed. If a mucocele is not seen in the nasal cavity then uncinectomy, anterior ethmoidectomy with identification of the skull base may need to be performed to gain access to the wall of the mucocele. A close scrutiny of the CT scan of the mucocele will help the surgeon to have proper exposure of the mucocele. Post-operative cavity care is the same as after any ethmoidectomy. The proptosis usually settles over a period of few weeks following surgery.

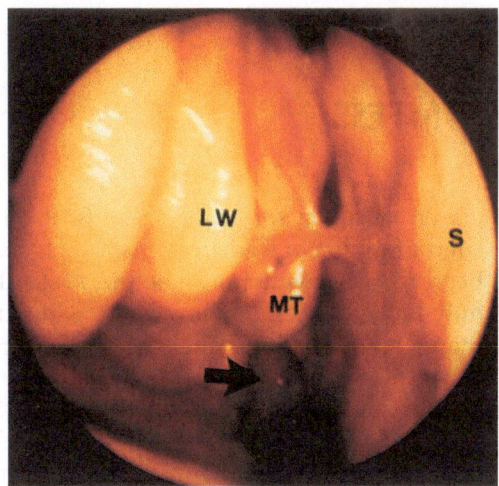

Fig. 15.10. Endoscopic view of the right nasal cavity in a patient who had had multiple sinus surgeries in the past. LW, prolapsed lateral wall of the nose with protrusion of the mucocele; MT, remnants of the middle turbinate; S, septum; post-nasal space (arrow).

Endoscopic Approach to Acute Sinusitis and Orbital Complications

Acute sinusitis most commonly responds to oral antibiotics and decongestants. However, there are cases in which the disease is disturbingly persistent and there is a further danger of infection spreading into the orbit or to the cranium.

The orbital complications such as orbital cellulitis and abscess most commonly arise from ethmoiditis. Patients who do not rapidly respond to intravenous antibiotics and decongestants need urgent surgical drainage. The problems during operation in acute cases are a congested and oedematous mucous membrane with vasodilatation and hence an increased tendency to bleed during operation. The surgical landmarks are distorted and there is an increased risk of complications, e.g. CSF leak during operation due to disease, inflammation and increased bleeding. Needless to emphasise that such an operation should only be undertaken by an experienced endoscopic surgeon (Fig. 11.7), otherwise an external approach should be performed for surgical drainage.

Chandler in 1970 proposed a classification of orbital complications of sinusitis as follows:

- inflammatory oedema
- orbital cellulitis
- subperiosteal abscess
- orbital abscess
- carvernous sinus thrombosis

The first three conditions are amenable to endoscopic ethmoidectomy and a surgical drainage; the last two, being more advanced and serious, should be approached by a combined technique of both endoscopic ethmoidectomy and an external ethmoid exploration and orbital decompression.

Lasers in FESS

Laser is an acronym for Light Amplification by Simulated Emission of Radiation. Although lasers have been used in medicine since the 1960s they have only recently been employed as a adjunct to endoscopic sinus surgery. Their action is three-fold: cutting, coagulation and vaporisation; all three actions are of use in FESS. The KTP/532 laser has the added advantage of fibre optic delivery systems, where the quartz fibre that transmits the laser energy can be passed through an endoscope, or a suitable hand-held instrument. This permits use of the laser right along the nasal cavity. The specific advantages of using KTP/532 in FESS are as follows:

- minimal bleeding, thereby allowing clear visualisation of surgical landmarks, making the surgery safe
- minimal trauma
- can be used under local anaesthetic
- green visible beam, therefore no need for an aiming beam as with other lasers
- as the KTP/532 wavelength is highly absorbed by the haemoglobin, it is a better coagulant.

Thus we find the KTP to be valuable for:

- nasal polyposis, where polyps could be evaporated with minimal bleeding

- adhesions, which can be divided with minimal risk of causing scar tissue
- using the property of "scatter" (dispersion of laser energy due to distance between the end of the probe and the target tissue), turbinate diathermy may be performed with minimum trauma to the surface lining, and maximum damage to the sub-mucosa
- evaporation of the posterior end of the inferior turbinate ("mulberry ends")
- excision of a concha bullosa
- wedge resection of middle turbinate

The disadvantages are:

- cost of equipment
- need for safety measures for all concerned as the laser gives out an extremely intense light, it can damage the retina. Hence, special glasses to filter the beam should be worn by all (including the patient).

We have so far performed 112 cases of endoscopic sinus surgery with KTP Laser, which included nasal polyposis, excision of concha bullosa, turbinoplasties, FESS revision cases, middle meatal antrostomies and excision of posterior ends of middle turbinates with great success.

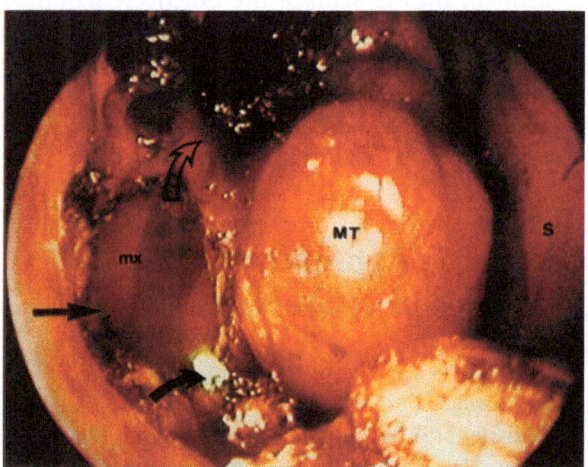

Fig. 15.11. Endoscopic view of a right revision FESS with a KTP/S32 laser. Straight arrow, middle meatal antrostomy; curved arrow, 600 micron quartz fibre transmitting laser creating a MMA; hollow curved arrow, ethmoid cavity, MT, middle turbinate; S, septum; MX, maxillary sinus.

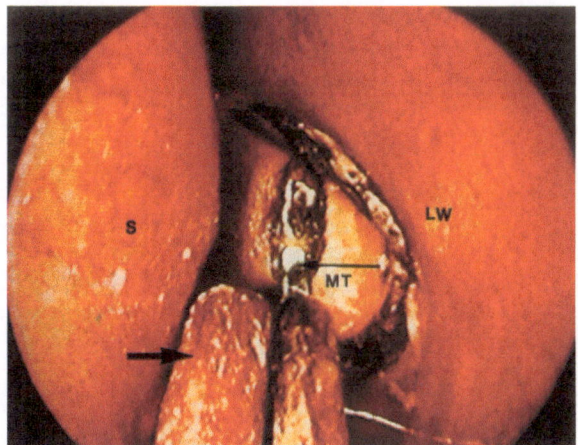

Fig. 15.12. Endoscopic view of the left nasal cavity during a KTP/S32 laser revision. FESS: excision of the anterior part of the middle turbinate. S, septum; MT, adherent middle turbinate to the lateral wall (LW) of the nose; thick arrow, suction part of the laser microstat long arrow, 600 micron quartz laser fibre. Note the complete absence of bleeding.

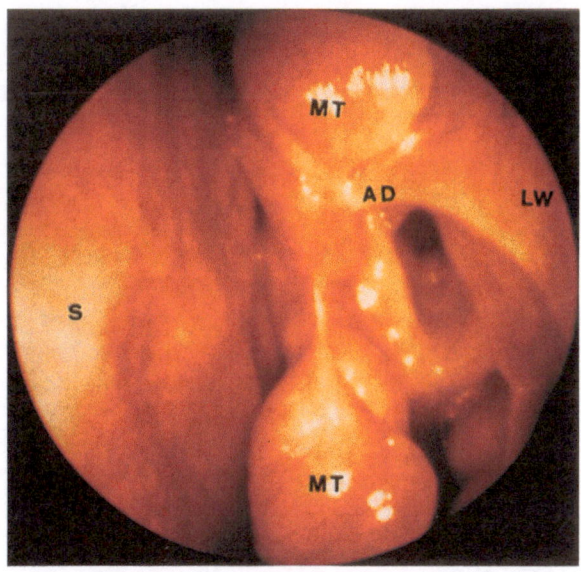

Fig. 15.14. Revision FESS: left nasal cavity. S, septum; MT, excised middle turbinate from previous surgery; LW, lateral wall; AD, adhesions between middle turbinate and lateral wall filling the ethmoid cavity.

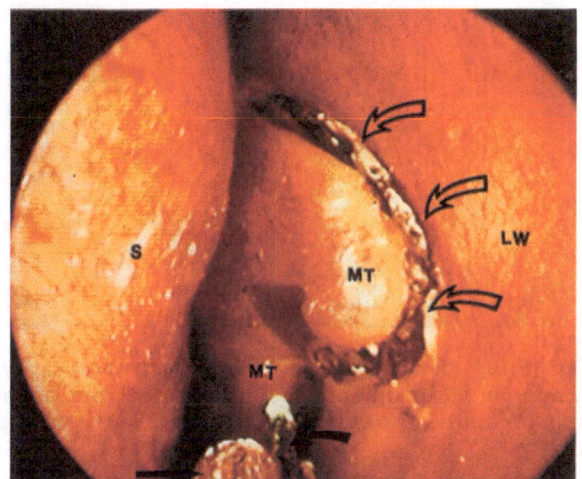

Fig. 15.13. Endoscopic view of the left nasal cavity showing KTP/S32 laser revision FESS. Laser uncinectomy has been performed (three hollow arrows). S, septum; MT, partially excised and adherent middle turbinate; straight arrow, suction part of the laser microstat; curved arrow, 600 micron quartz fibre transmitting laser.

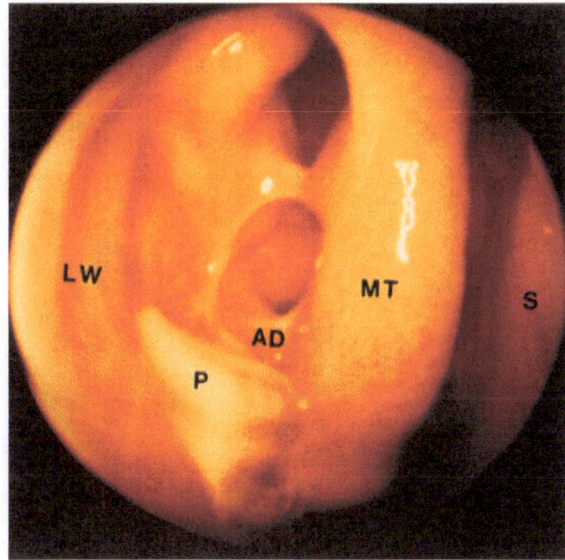

Fig. 15.15. Revision FESS: right nasal cavity. AD, adhesions between the middle turbinate (MT) and the lateral wall (LW) filling the ethmoid cavity; P, pus exuding from the maxillary sinus; S, septum.

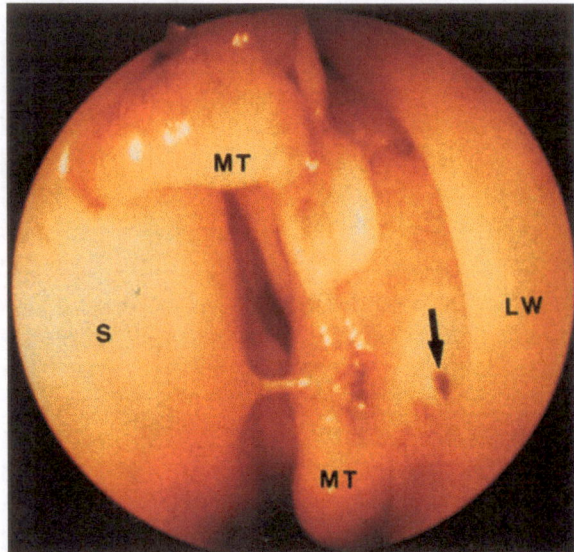

Fig. 15.16. Revision FESS: left nasal cavity. S, septum; MT, remnants of the middle turbinate following two previous sinus operations; LW, lateral wall; arrow shows stenosed middle meatal nasal antrostomy.

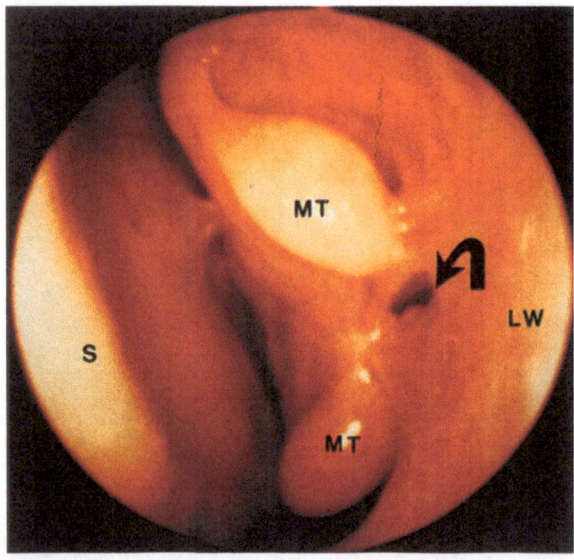

Fig. 15.17. Revision FESS: Left nasal cavity. S, septum; MT, middle turbinate adherent to the lateral wall (LW) after previous partial excision; arrow shows stenosed middle meatal antrostomy.

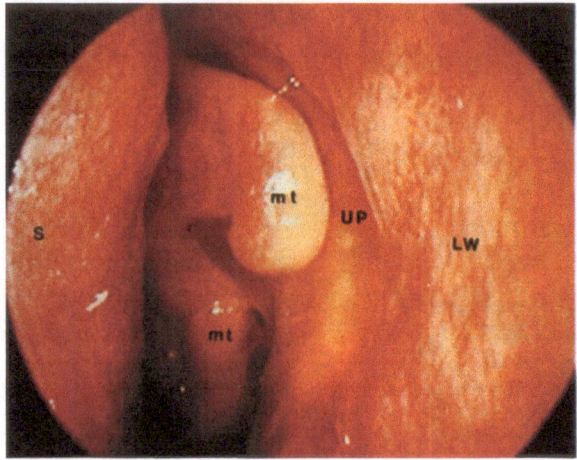

Fig. 15.18. Revision FESS: left side of nasal cavity. S, septum; MT, middle turbinate partially excised and adherent to the lateral wall (LW); UP, uncinate process.

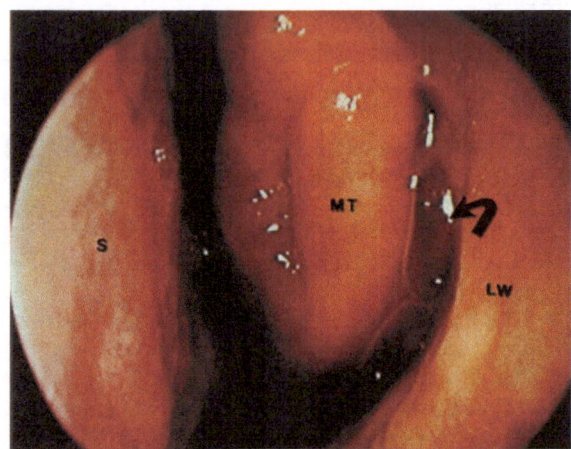

Fig. 15.19. Revision surgery: left side of nasal cavity. S, septum; MT, middle turbinate adherent to the lateral wall (LW); arrow shows polypoidal disease in the middle meatus.

Endoscopic Orbital Decompression

Orbital decompression for dysthyroid orbitopathy has been performed in the past either through the antrum or externally. With the advent of intranasal endoscopes it is now possible to decompress the medial and inferior wall of the orbit, thereby relieving pressure on the optic nerve. This clearly avoids the morbidity of the external ethmoidectomy or Caldwell-Luc antrotomy.

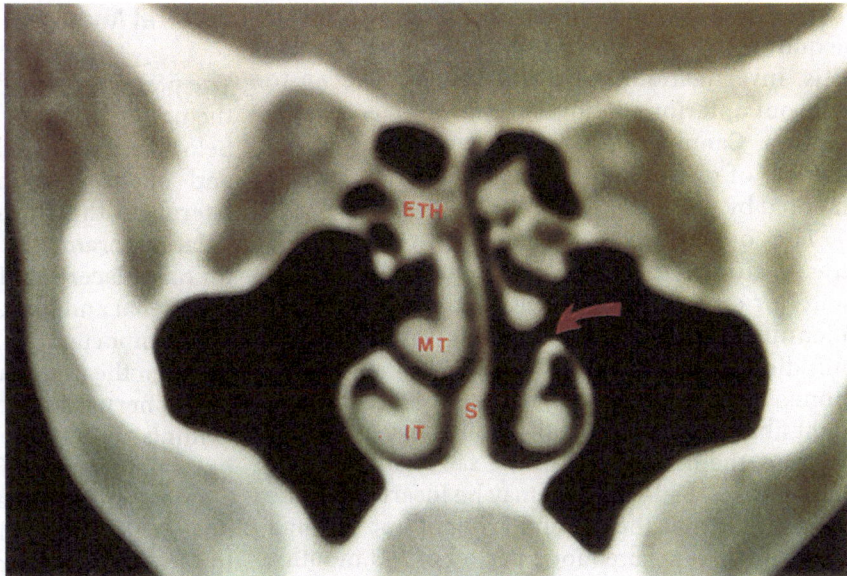

Fig. 15.20. Revision FESS. Coronal CT scan showing mucosal disease in the posterior ethmoid sinuses (ETH); middle turbinate (MT); septum (S); inferior turbinate (IT); middle meatal antrostomy (arrow).

Endoscopic orbital decompression is performed under general anaesthesia. A complete sphenoethmoidectomy is performed to skeletonize the medial wall of the orbit and the skull base. Anteriorly the frontal recess and posteriorly the orbital apex are identified. A large middle meatal antrostomy is performed from the posterior margin of the nasolacrimal duct anteriorly to the posterior limit of the maxillary sinus. Inferiorly the antrostomy extends to the attachment of the inferior turbinate. The exposed medial wall of the orbit is then removed with a blunt hook or similar instrument. The lateral limit for the removal of the bone of the orbital floor is the position of the infraorbital nerve seen through the large antrostomy. Care is taken to preserve the small bony area of the medial wall of the orbit near the frontal recess or else the soft tissues will obstruct the frontal recess.

When removal of the bony orbital wall is complete, the periorbita is incised with a sickle knife in linear strokes from posterior to the anterior. Further fibrous periorbital bands are excised to allow the orbital contents to prolapse into the maxillary sinus and into the nasal cavity. The extent of decompression is assessed by palpating the eyeball and looking for herniated orbital contents in the nose through the endoscope. The post-operative care is same as for any other sphenoethmoidectomy.

Endoscopic Dacryocystorhinostomy (DCR)

As the endoscope broadens our horizons, it leads us to a structure that is traditionally within the purview of the ophthalmologist, the orbit. When one considers that two out of the three walls of the eye socket abut the nasal and sinus cavities, procedures involving this structure can logically also be handled by the otolaryngologist. Endoscopic control allows for tackling disease at the lower end of the naso-lacrimal apparatus, which is the most common site of affection. It has made the technique an even more aesthetic and successful procedure in the hands of the ear, nose and throat surgeon. Furthermore, an anterior ethmoid focus of disease may be tackled simultaneously. Indeed, a significant number of dacryocystitis cases are caused by infection in the anterior ethmoidal cells.

The advantages include:

■ internal approach; therefore no external incision

■ can be performed under local anaesthesia (day-case surgery)

■ good success rate comparable with the external approach

The operation is performed for a congenital or acquired stenosis, producing chronic dacryocystitis. Investigations include a coronal CT scan to rule out anterior ethmoid disease and dacryocystogram. Cannulation is then performed to locate the site of obstruction; it may be further supplemented by a retinal light probe.

The operation is performed by an initial uncinectomy, followed by exenteration of the anterior ethmoidal cells. The lacrimal sac is then identified just in front of the anterior end of the middle turbinate, by removing the overlying bone. The sac may be illuminated by passing a light fibre along the inferior canaliculus. Once this is done, the medial wall of the sac is excised and left open, or a silastic tube may be inserted via the canaliculus into the sac and brought out through the nose to be secured for a period of 2–3 months. Published reports suggest excellent results with minimum morbidity and complications.

Vidian Neurectomy

This operation is based on the fact that the autonomic nerve supply to the nasal cavity is through sympathetic and parasympathetic fibres, carried by the vidian nerve. The vidian nerve is formed from the union of pre-ganglionic parasympathetic fibres from the greater superficial petrosal nerve with post-ganglionic fibres containing the deep petrosal nerve. The nerve runs across the pterygo-palatine fossa to connect with the spheno-palatine ganglion, from where post-ganglionic parasympathetic fibres emerge to supply the nasal mucosa. They exert their action via the release of acetylcholine.

Vasomotor instability is manifested mainly by rhinorrhea, excessive sneezing, nasal obstruction and headaches. Rhinorrhea is the most characteristic symptom, and is due to excessive overactivity of the seromucinous glands. This, together with increased capillary permeability and vascular dilatation results in copious, clear and watery secretions of low mucin content. Nasal obstruction occurs because of enormous dilatation and oedema of the inferior turbinate. Headaches follow because of insufficient ventilation. Racial, constitutional and emotional factors play an important part in the aetiology of this condition.

Surgical Anatomy

The pterygoid or vidian canal is bounded above by the undersurface of the body of the sphenoid, and below by the medial pterygoid plate. The anterior end opens into the pterygo-maxillary fissure, lateral to the posterior border of the spheno-palatine foramen. Its posterior end opens into the foramen lacerum. The nerve traverses the pterygoid canal and joins the spheno-palatine ganglion. It is important to note that the ganglion lies between the mucosa and the periosteum, while the vidian nerve lies between the periosteum and bone (Minnis, 1971). The average distance between the posterior border of the septum and the anterior opening of the vidian canal is 18.6 mm, while the distance from the mouth of the vidian canal to the foramen rotundum is 6.5 mm. The distance between the pterygoid canal from the posterior border of the spheno-palatine foramen is 2 mm. The average dimensions of the pterygoid canal are 1.5–2.5 mm diameter and 19–20 mm length.

Vidian neurectomy has been a well-established procedure in the treatment of vasomotor rhinitis. Several routes to the vidian nerve have been described, including the trans-antral, trans-palatal and trans-nasal. The endoscope may be used to access the spheno-palatine foramen and thereby the pterygoid canal via the trans-nasal route.

Technique

Under general anaesthetic, a 4 mm angled (30°) endoscope is used to visualise the posterior end of the middle turbinate, which may need lateralisation to allow better access. The mouth of the spheno-palatine foramen is then located by one of three methods (Khasgiwala 1972):

- just posterior to or slightly above the posterior end of the middle turbinate

- at the junction of the superior and lateral walls of the nasal cavity, 12–14 mm antero-superior to the superior border of the posterior choana

- the superior turbinate acts as a "pointer" to the spheno-palatine foramen

The site of the foramen is confirmed with an insulated, 15 cm blunt probe, and an incision is made over the posterior (relatively avascular) lip with a sickle knife. The muco-periosteum is dissected forwards to expose the foramen under endoscopic control. The spheno-palatine artery is often encountered here; however, it rarely bleeds as it has its own covering and may be kept away from the operative field. The probe is further advanced into the foramen in a posterior direction, thus separating the periosteum off the lateral wall of the sphenoid process of the palatine bone. The opening of the pterygoid canal is reached 5–6 mm posterior and lateral to the spheno-palatine foramen. Finally, a slim cautery/probe is inserted into the dissected foramen and used to cauterise the vidian nerve. The mucosa is then replaced; no packing is normally necessary. Both sides are done at one sitting.

The procedure is a distinct step forward from the gross or microscopic trans-nasal approaches, as it allows for angled visualisation of the lateral nasal wall, and better visualisation of the pterygo-palatine foramen. Some published results show a high degree of efficacy of the technique.

Appendix

Appendix A. Instruments

Instruments Used in Office Nasal Endoscopy

1. Hopkins straight telescope, 0°, 4 mm, fibre optic light transmission incorporated
2. Hopkins forward oblique telescope, 30°, 4 mm
3. Cold Light Fountain, 220 VAC, 40–60 Hz.
   150 watt halogen lamp
   colour temperature approximately 3400 K
   with two light outlets
   light intensity adjustable
4. Fibre optic light cable, size 3.5 mm, length 230 cm
5. Wittmoser Articulated Optical Arm with 4 joints, length 820 mm. Used for optically connecting the endoscopic telescope through a still or video camera, and for simultaneous observation by the operator and observer
6. Special zoom lens with adapter to Hopkins telescope for still photography

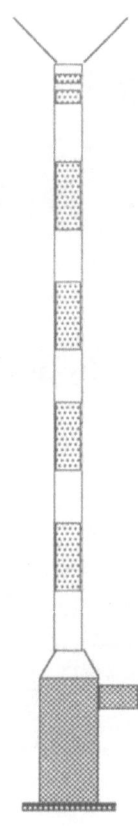

Fig. A.1. The Hopkins rod lens system affords a smaller diameter, a larger viewing angle and a brighter image.

Instruments Used in FESS

1. Hopkins straight telescope, 0°, 4 mm, fibre optic light transmission incorporated
2. Hopkins forward oblique telescope, 30°, 4 mm
3. Hopkins wide-angle lateral telescope, 70°, 4 mm
4. Hopkins wide-angle lateral telescope, 2.7 mm, 0°
5. Hopkins wide-angle lateral telescope, 2.7 mm, 30°
6. Anti-fog solution
7. Endoscope sleeve (for good grip and precision of movements)

8. Killian's fibre optic nasal speculum, 7.5 cm
9. Freer elevator, double ended, 20 cm
10. Angular long needle (for local anaesthetic)
11. Sickle knife, 19 cm, pointed
12. Blakesly Weil ethmoid forceps, 19 cm, size No. 1, size No. 4
13. Blakesly Weil ethmoid forceps, upturned, 19 cm, size No.2
14. Blakesly Weil ethmoid forceps, upturned, 90°, size No.2 (for frontal recess and middle meatal antrostomy)

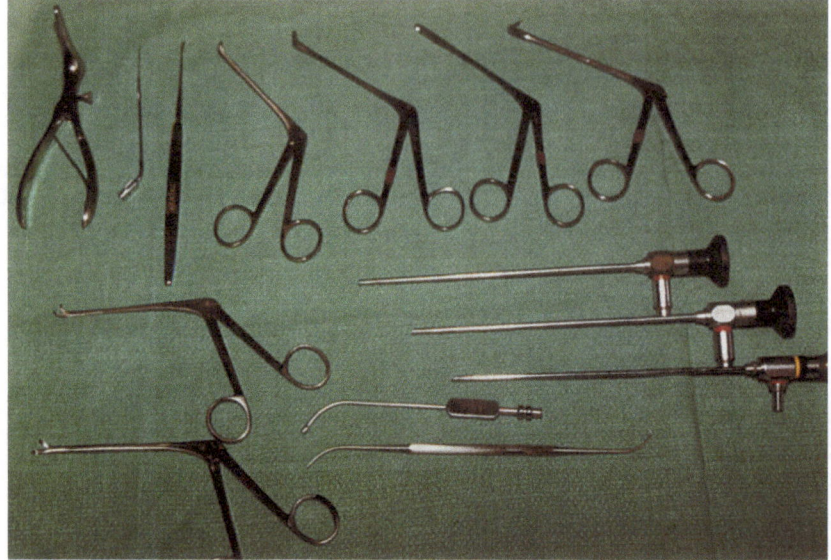

Fig. A.2. Instrument set commonly used for FESS. Top, from left to right: Killian's fibre optic speculum, endoscopic needle, sickle knife, small and large 45° upward-cutting forceps, straight forceps, backward-cutting forceps. Bottom, from left to right: "cut through" straight and upward-cutting forceps, suction cannula, maxillary and frontal ostium seeker, three 4-mm endoscopes (0°, 30° and 70°).

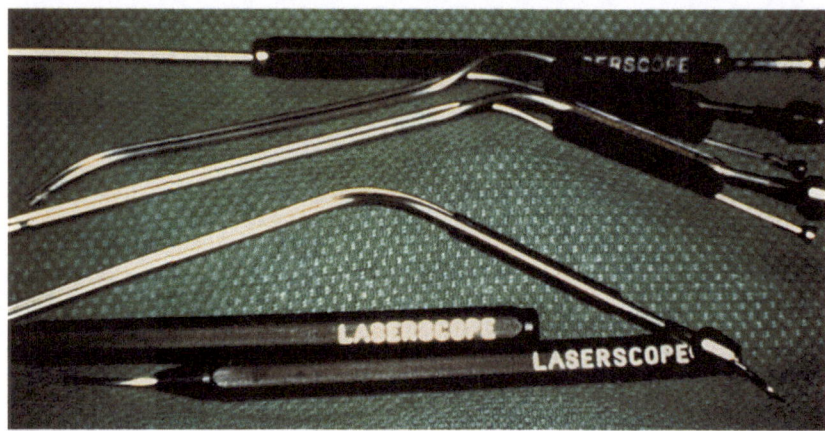

Fig. A.3. A set of KTP 532 laser delivery instruments for endoscopic sinus surgery.

15. Stammberger backward-cutting forceps (for middle meatal antrostomy)
16. Endoscopic scissors
17. Angled suction
18. Trocar and cannula (for maxillary sinoscopy)
19. Giraffe forceps

Care of Instruments

Endoscopy instruments are expensive, and should be handled with care! All steel instruments can be autoclaved. The endoscopes and fibre optic cables are chemically sterilised with CIDEX, although autoclavable endoscopes have recently became available.

Appendix B. Documentation

Proforma

In order to keep accurate records of all our patients, we developed computer-compatible proformas for pre-, intra- and post-operative notes. The proformas also display key areas visually, in order to give the surgeon a rough pictorial representation of the disease. The graphic on Chart 2, for example, depicts the site and extent of disease which could then be accurately monitored post-operatively. Each piece of information is given a number, so that it may be processed on a database.

Functional Endoscopic Sinus Surgery Chart (1)

Age _____ years
Sex   0   (male)
         1   (female)

Consultant - S.K. Kaluskar, M.S.,F.R.C.S.,D.L.O.(Eng.)
Tyrone County Hospital, Omagh, Northern Ireland

Catalogue number [9 /]

name _____

address _____
_____
_____

Date of operation ____|____|____

Surgeon / s   — — — — — — — —
Anaesthetist   — — — — — — — —

hosp. no. _____

d.o.birth _____
sticker if available

Pre-Operative Assessment

Grades:
1 - mild, 2 - moderate, 3 - severe

Symptoms
nasal obstruction

2,3,4	R / L / bilateral
5,6,7	Grade: 1 2 3

asthma   16
ASA intolerance   17

post-nasal drip

8,9,10	Grade: 1 2 3

headaches & facial pains

11,12,13	Grade: 1 2 3

allergic profile
18,19,20 Grade : 1 2 3
   21   sneezing
   22   rhinorrhea
   23   nasal irritation

h/o allergies   Y/N   14,15
allergens _____

Anterior Rhinoscopy
septal deviation

31,32,33	-	R / L / bilateral
34,35	-	caudal / high

polyps

36,37,38	-	R / L / bilateral
39,40	-	single / multiple

smell
anosmia   24
hyposmia   25
parosmia   26

misc.
sore throats   27
laryngitis   28
LRTI   29
otitis media   30

N. Endoscopy

high septal deviation - R / L / bilateral	41,42,43

Sphe.- eth.
recess   57a

uncinate process (R / L)	44,45
- concha bullosa (R / L) / paradoxical turb. (R / L)	46,47,48,49

Acc. Os   57b

- bulla ethmoidales (R / L) / agger nasi (R / L)	50,51,52,53
- m. meatus : polyps (R / L) / mucopus (a / p)	54,55,56,57

Past History

- Caldwell Luc / IN Antrostomy / Polypectomy /	58,59,60,
Sinusitis / Chest Complaints	61,62

Functional Endoscopic Sinus Surgery Chart ②

Plain Xrays	grade R/L	cyst / fl. level R/L	
maxillary			63
frontal			to
ethmoid			78
sphenoid			

clear 0, slight haziness 1, marked haziness 2

CT scan	grade R/L	other R/L	
maxillary			79
frontal			to
ethmoid			94
sphenoid			

clear 0, haziness 1

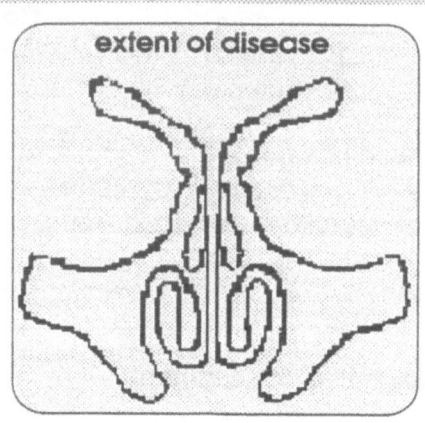

extent of disease

key areas on CT scan

Rt.   Lt.

u.p.
bulla ethmoidales
ethmoid infundibulum
m.t.
frontal recess
ant. eth.
post.eth. 95 to 106
sphenoid
fovea eth.
l.p.
o.n.(O.cell)
ica

Additional Remarks :

Operative Notes
- **LA / GA**   107, 108
- unilateral / bilateral   109, 110

approach
- nasal / combined   111, 112

ethmoidectomy   113, 114
- anterior / frn.sinusotomy / mma
- posterior / sphenoidotomy / fro.sin./mma
                                115, 116
Mx. ostium   117, 118
- blocked - thick muco. / polyps / granu.

-**sinus mucosa**   119, 120
  nor. / thick. / polypoidal / cysts 121, 122

- **associated procedures**
- septo / rhinoplasty -   123, 124
- ear   125

- **any complications**   126

POST OP. FOLLOW UP

no change 1, mild improvement 2, good improvement 3, no sym.4
nasal endoscopy : well healed 1, disease present 2

follow - up	3 mon.	6 mon.	1 yr.	18 mon.	2 yr.	3 yr.	4 yr.	5 yr.
nasal obst.								
P.N.D.								
headaches - f.pain								

SKK / ASK

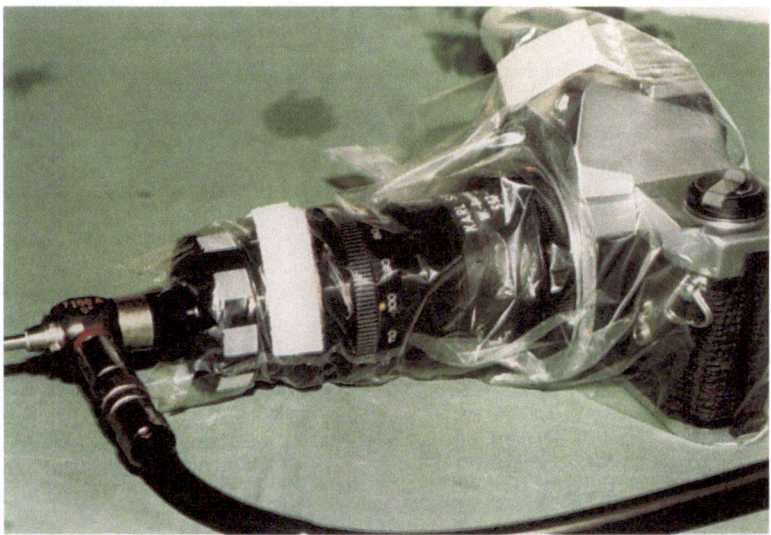

Fig. A.4. Single Lens Reflex camera with a special zoom lens for endoscopic still photography.

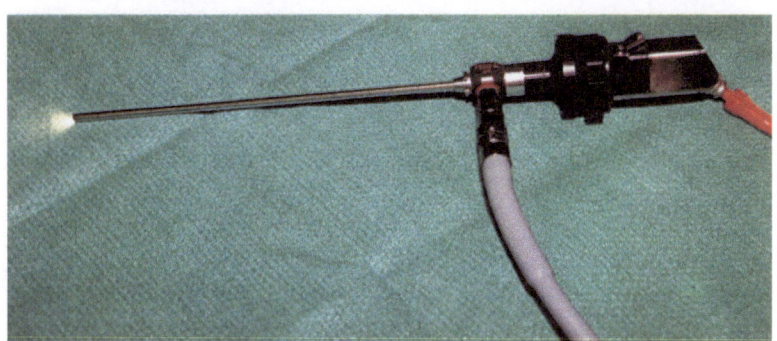

Fig. A.5. A 4-mm 0° endoscopic CCD video camera with C-mount.

Still Photography

1. Single lens reflex camera
2. Zoom lens, f 70–140, with adapter to Hopkins telescope
3. Cold light fountain, 150 or 250 watt
4. Ektachrome slide daylight film (high-quality prints may be made)
5. Customised sterile camera drape (for intra-operative photography)

Video Photography

1. CCD video camera
2. High resolution colour monitor
3. Super VHS video recorder
4. Pro-grade S-VHS video tapes
5. Professional editing suite with high-resolution monitors using a Commodore Amiga with title software

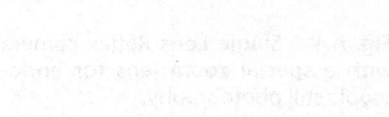

Bibliography

Anderson I, Camner P, Jenson PL, Philipson K, Proctor DF (1974) A comparison of nasal and tracheobronchial clearance. Arch Environ Health 29: 290–293

Aust R, Drettner B (1974a) The functional size of the human maxillary ostium in vivo. Acta Otolaryngol 78: 432–435

Aust R, Drettner B (1974b) Oxygen tension in human maxillary sinus under normal and pathological conditions. Acta Otolaryngol 78: 264–269

Berthon E (1880) Essai sur less abcés et hydropiris des sinus frontaux. Thesis, Paris

Bryant FL (1960) Management of chronic maxillary sinusitis in children. J La State Med Soc 112: 390–393

Buiter CT (1976) Endoscopy of the upper airway. Elsevier, Amsterdam

Buiter CT, Straatman NJA (1981) Endoscopic antrostomy in the nasal fontanelle. Rhinology 19: 17–24

Chandler JR, Langenbrunaer DJ, Stevens ER (1970) The pathogenesis of orbital complications and acute sinusitis. Laryngoscope 80: 1414–1428

Dedola GL (1987) Computed tomography of the ethmoid labyrinth and adjacent structures. Ann Otol Rhinol Laryngol 96: 239–250

Deitmer TH (1989) Physiology and pathology of mucociliary system. Adv 43 Otorhinolaryngol

Dezeimeris, cited by Berthon (1880)

Draf W (1978) Endoscopy of the paranasal sinuses. Actas, XI World Congress for ORL, Buenos Aires

Draf W (1982) Die chirurgische Behandlung entzündlicher Erkrankungen der Nasennebenhöhlen. Arch Otorhinolaryngol 235: 133–305, 367–377

Draf W (1983) Endoscopy of the paranasal sinuses. Springer, Berlin Heidelberg New York

Evert G (1965) On the mucous flow rate in the human nose. Acta Otolaryngol (Stockh) [Suppl] 200: 1

Fairbanks DFN (1986) Complications of nasal packing. Otolaryngol Head Neck Surg 94: 412–415

Fawcett D, Porter K (1954) Study of the fine structure of ciliated epithelia. J Morphol 94: 221

Flottes L, Clerc P, Riu R, Devilla F (1960) La physiologie des sinus. Libraire Arnette, Paris

Ginzel A, Ellum P (1980) Nasal mucociliary clearance in patients with septal deviation. Rhinology 18: 177–181

Grünwald L (1925) Deskriptive und topographische Anatomie der Nase und ihrer Nebenhöhlen In: Denker A, Kahler O (eds) Handbuch der Hals-Nasen-Ohrenheilkunde. Springer, Berlin Heidelberg New York, pp 1–95

Hackett F (1934) Francis I. Doubleday, New York, 613–616

Hady MRA, Shehata O, Hassan R (1983) Nasal mucociliary function in different diseases of the nose. J Laryngol Otol 97: 497–502

Hansen R (1968) Headaches of nasal origin. Laryngoscope 78: 1164–1171

Hara MJ (1962) Severe epistaxis. Arch Otolaryngol Head Neck Surg 75: 258–269

Harper OV, Andros G, Lathrop KA (1962) Observation on the use of 6 hours 99^m technetium as a tracer in biology and medicine. Argonne Cancer Res Hosp 18: 76–80

Herrnheisser G (1926) Der Rontegenbefund bei der mucocele oder pycele der Stirnhohle und der Siebbeinzellen. Z Hals Nasen 14: 319–326

Hilding AC (1931) Ciliary activity and course of secretion currents of the nose. Proc Mayo Clin 6: 285

Hilding AC (1932) Physiology of drainage of nasal mucous: experimental work on accessory sinuses. Am J Physiol 100: 664

Hilding AC (1941) Experimental sinus surgery: effects of operation windows on normal sinuses. Ann Otol Rhinol Laryngol 50: 379–392

Hilding AC (1944) The role of ciliary action in production of pulmonary atelectasis, vacuum in the paranasal sinuses, and in otitis media. Ann Otol 52: 816–833

Hilding AC (1950) Physiologic basis of nasal operations. Calif Med 72: 103–107

Howarth WC (1921) Mucocele and pyocele of the accessory nasal sinuses. Lancet II: 744–746

Illum P, Jeppesen F (1972) Sinoscopy: endoscopy of the maxillary sinus. Technique, common and rare findings. Acta Otolaryngol [Stockh.] 73: 506–512

Jakus MA, Hall CE (1946) Electron microscope observations of trichocysts and cilia of paramecium. Biol Bull 91: 131–146

Jensen PF, Kristensen S, Juul A, Johannessen NW (1991) Episodic nocturnal hypoxia and nasal packing. Clin Otolaryngol 16: 433–435

Kaluskar SK, Patil NP (1992a) The role of out-patient nasal endoscopy in the evaluation of chronic sinus disease. (editorial). Clin Otolaryngol 17: 193–194

Kaluskar SK, Patil NP (1992b) Combined approach middle meatal antrostomy (CAMMA) Laryngoscope 102: 709–711

Kaluskar SK, Patil NP (1992c) Clinical atlas of ear, nose and throat diseases. Bhalani Publishing House, India

Kaluskar SK, Patil NP (1992d) Office nasal endoscopy in the evaluation of chronic sinus disease. Karl Storz

Kaluskar SK, Patil NP, Sharkey AN (1993) The role of CT in functional endoscopic sinus surgery. Rhinology 31: 49–52

Kaluskar SK, Leydon P (1994) Endoscopic approach to posterior epistaxis. Proc Irish Otolaryngol Soc 1994: 39–42

Kaluskar SK (1995) Endoscopic approach to orbital complications. Presented at Functional Endoscopic Sinus Surgery Meeting, April 1995, Omagh, N. Ireland

Kaluskar SK (1995) KTP/532 Laser in Functional Endoscopic Sinus Surgery. Presented at Advanced Symposium on Sinus Surgery, August 1995, Cairns, Australia

Kaluskar SK (1996) KTP/532 Laser in Revision Endoscopic Sinus Surgery. Presented at World Association of Laser Therapy, June 1996, Jerusalem, Israel

Kaluskar SK (1996) Endoscopic approach to posterior epistaxis. J Min Invasive Ther All Technol 5: 75–77

Karenfelt C, et al. (1978) The role of local gas composition in pathogenesis of maxillary sinus empyema Acta Otolaryngol 85: 116–121

Kennedy DW, Goodstein ML, Miller NR, Zinreich SJ (1990) Endoscopic transnasal orbital decompression. Arch Otolaryngol Head Neck Surg 116: 275–282

Khasgiwala CK (1972) Vidian neurocoagulation via transseptal approach. MS thesis, University of Gujarat, India

King E (1935) A clinical study of the functioning of the maxillary sinus mucosa. Ann Otol 44: 480–482

Langenbeck CJM (1819) Neue Bibliohek fur die Chirugie and opthalmologie. Bey DanBrudern Hahn, Hannover

Langraf-Favre FF (1974) Pain of nasal origin. Rhinology 12: 73–78

Lynch RC (1921) The technique of a radical frontal sinus operation which has given me the best results. 31: 1–5

Mattox DE, Kennedy DW (1990) Endoscopic management of cerebrospinal fluid leaks and cephaloceles. Laryngoscope 100: 857–862

McGarry GW (1991) Nasal endoscope in posterior epistaxis, a preliminary evaluation. J Laryngol Otol 105: 428–431

Messerklinger W (1978) Endoscopy of the nose. Urban & Schwarzenberg, Munich

Mosher HP (1912) The applied anatomy and the intranasal surgery of the ethmoidal labyrinth. Trans Am Laryngol Assoc 34: 25–39

Mosher HP (1929) The surgical anatomy of the ethmoidal labyrinth. Am Acad Ophthalmol Otolaryngol 376–410

Myerson MC (1932) The natural orifice of the maxillary sinus. Anatomic Studies. Arch Otolaryngol 15: 80–91

O'Leary, Stickney K, Makielski K, Weymuller EA Jr (1992) Rigid endoscopy for the control of epistaxis. Arch Otolaryngol Head Neck Surg 118: 966–967

Onodi A (1901) Das Verhaltniss der kieferhole zurkeilbein hohle und zu der vorderen Siebbeinzellen. Arch Laryngol Rhinol 11: 391–395

Proctor DF, Wagner HN (1965) Clearance of particles from the human nose. Arch Environ Health 11: 366–371

Proetz AW (1941) Essays on the applied physiology of the nose. Annals Publ. St Louis

Puchelle E, Aug F, Zahm JN, Bertrand A (1981) Comparison of three methods for measuring nasal mucociliary clearance in man. Acta Otolaryngol 91: 247–303

Quinlan M, Salmon S, Swift D, Wagner H, Proctor DF (1969) Measurement of mucociliary function in man. Am Rev Respir Dis 99: 13

Rogers JH (1976) Mucocele of the paranasal sinuses. Otolaryngol Clin North Am 9: 233

Rollet M (1896) Mucocele de l'angle superointern des orbites. Lyon Med 81: 573–575

Rollet M (1909) In: Lagrange F, Valude E (eds) Encyclopedie francaise d'opthalmology. Doin, Paris, 588

Ryan RE et al. (1979) Headache of nasal origin. Headache 19: 173–179

Sakakura Y, Majuma Y, Saida S, Ukai K, Mioshi Y (1985) Reversibility of reduced mucociliary clearance in chronic sinusitis. Clin Otolaryngol 10: 79–83

Shaheen OH (1975) Arterial epistaxis. J Laryngol Otol 89: 17

Sluder G (1927) Nasal neurology: headache and eye disorders. Kimpton, London 1927

Stammberger H (1985) Endoscopic surgery for mycotic and chronic recurring sinusitis. Ann Otol Rhinol Laryngol 94 (suppl 119): 1–11

Stammberger H (1986a) Nasal and paranasal sinus endoscopy: a diagnostic and surgical approach to recurrent sinusitis. Endoscopy 6: 213–218

Stammberger H (1986b) Endoscopic endonasal surgery: concepts in treatment of recurring rhinosinusitis. 1. Anatomic and pathophysiologic considerations. 11. Technique. Otolaryngol Head Neck Surg 94: 143–156

Stammberger H, Zinreich SJ, Kopp W, Kennedy DW, Johns ME, Rosenbaum AE (1987) Zur operativen Behandlung der chronisch-rezidivierenden Sinusitis – Caldwell-Luc versus funktionelle endoskopische Technik. Head Neck Otolaryngol 35: 93–105

Terrier G, Baumann RP, Pidoux JM (1976) Endoscopic and histopathological observations of chronic maxillary sinusitis. Rhinology 14: 129–132

Tremble GE (1948) Clinical observations in movement of nasal cilia. Laryngoscope 206–224

Waitz G, Wigand ME (1992) Results of endoscopic sinus surgery for the treatment of inverted papillomas. Laryngoscope 102: 917–922

Wang et al. (1981) Posterior epistaxis. Comparison of treatment. Otolaryngol Head Neck Surg 89: 1001–1006

Weiss N (1990) Otolaryngology: an illustrated history. Butterworth, London

Weiss NS (1972) Relation of high blood pressure to headache epistaxis, and selected other symptoms. N Engl J Med 287: 631

Wigand ME (1981) Transnasal ethmoidectomy under endoscopical control. Rhinology 19: 7–15

Wigand ME, Hosemann W (1985) Endoscopic ethmoidectomy for chronic sinubronchitis. In: Myers E (ed) New dimensions in otorhinolaryngology: head and neck surgery, vol. 1. Elsevier, Amsterdam, pp 549–552

Wigand ME, Steiner W, Jaumann MP (1978) Endonasal sinus surgery with endoscopical control: from radical operation to rehabilitation of the mucosa. Endoscopy 10: 255–260

Woodruff GH (1949) Cardiovascular epistaxis and the nasopharyngeal plexus. Laryngoscope 59: 1238–1247

Wurman LH, Garry Sack J, Flannery JV, Paulson TO (1988) Selective endoscopic electrocautery for posterior epistaxis. Laryngoscope 98: 1348–1349

Wurman LH, Sack JG, Flannery JV Jr, Lipsman RA (1992) The management of epistaxis. Am J Otolaryngol 193–209

Zinreich SJ, Kennedy DW, Rosenbaum AE, Gayler BW, Kumar AJ, Stammberger H (1987) CT of nasal cavity and paranasal sinuses: imaging requirements for functional endoscopic sinus surgery. J Radiol 163: 769–775

Zizmor J (1974) Mucocele of the paranasal sinuses, Can J Otolaryngol [Suppl] 1

Index

A

Agger Nasi   7, 9, 13, 22, 26, 27, 61, 76, 77, 94, 98
Allergy   15, 49
Anaesthesia   51, 52
Antibiotics   48, 71
Antrochoanal polyp   13, 25
Anterior ethmoidal artery   84, 85, 87, 89

B

Bulla ethmoidales   4, 9, 10, 11, 22, 28, 29, 34, 37, 38, 44, 54, 55, 60, 61

C

Calwell Luc   2, 65
CAMMA   60, 61, 63
Canine fossa   63
Cilia   16, 17, 18
Concha bullosa (conchal sinus)   10, 12, 22, 39, 43, 58, 65, 67, 76, 77, 97, 98
Corticosteroids   48
Cribriform plate   12, 36, 38, 39, 43, 44, 59, 83, 84, 85, 88
Crista galli   5, 11, 36, 37, 38, 43, 68
CSF   83, 84, 87, 107, 113

D

DCR   107
Developmental anatomy of nose   3

E

Ecchymosis   68, 79, 80, 81, 82, 100
Epiphora   100, 112
Epistaxis   100, 107, 108
Eustachian tube   3, 21, 24, 25, 29, 56, 108

F

FEONA   35, 36
Fontanelle   9, 13, 19, 58, 60, 80
Frontal recess   7, 10, 11, 13, 36, 38, 56, 60, 61, 68, 69

G

Ground lamella   11, 12, 22, 29, 34, 40, 57, 59, 72, 73, 80, 94

H

Haller cells   34, 37, 43, 77
Hiatus semilunaris   4, 7, 9, 10, 11, 22

I

Inferior meatal antrostomy (IMA)   21, 24, 38, 66
Inferior meatus   7, 21
Infundibular block   34
Infundibulum   7, 10, 11, 13, 36, 38, 39, 42, 43, 57, 60, 62
Internal carotid artery   5, 33, 59, 79, 90, 104

L

Lacrimal sac   117
Lacrimal bone   7, 55
Lamina papyracea   5, 10, 11, 12, 29, 33, 34, 35, 37, 38, 42, 43, 55, 57, 59, 71, 80, 82, 84, 85, 87, 95, 96
Lateral nasal wall   8, 9, 11, 25, 26, 27, 28, 29, 30, 53, 54, 57, 58, 59, 72, 73, 113, 115
Laser   114, 115

M

Medial rectus   5, 37, 40, 79, 104, 113
Middle meatal antrostomy   58, 59, 60, 61, 71, 73, 80, 83, 94, 95, 116, 117
Middle meatus   4, 7, 9, 27, 34, 51, 52

N

Nasolacrimal duct   7, 11, 21, 79, 80

O

Ostio-meatal complex   9, 15, 21, 27, 33, 37, 49, 60, 65, 67, 76

Optic foramen   6
Optic nerve   5, 11, 33, 35, 40, 55, 56, 59, 79, 82, 89
Orbit   4, 33, 34, 57, 83
Ostium   17, 26, 27, 28
   accessory   10, 11, 13, 19, 22, 25, 28, 29, 58, 60, 61
   natural (maxillary)   4, 7, 9, 11, 13, 19, 22, 59, 60, 61, 62,
      75, 77
   sphenoidal   22, 29, 30, 31

P

Para-infundibular block   35
Pneumatisation   58, 62, 65, 76
Proforma   122, 123, 124

S

Saccharin   18, 68
Sinusitis, bacteriology   48
Skull base (anterior cranial fossa)   4, 5, 33, 55, 56, 57, 59,
      60, 61, 71, 83, 104
Sphenoethmoidal recess   7, 12, 22, 29
Sphenopalatine artery   79, 80
Superior meatus   7, 12
Synaechiae (adhesions)   31, 71, 79, 83, 100

T

Turbinates   3, 4, 5, 7, 8, 75
   inferior   3, 4, 5, 7, 8, 11, 12, 13, 23, 25, 28, 29, 37, 39, 40,
      44, 57, 59, 60, 72, 73
   middle   3, 4, 5, 7, 8, 11, 12, 13, 19, 22, 23, 25, 26, 27, 28,
      29, 30, 31, 36, 37, 38, 39, 40, 42, 43, 44, 57, 65, 76,
      92, 93, 115, 116
   superior   7, 8, 11, 22, 28, 29, 30, 31, 38, 41, 42, 43, 44,
      56, 76
   supreme   7, 11

U

Uncinate process   4, 9, 10, 11, 12, 13, 22, 28, 29, 34, 36,
      37, 38, 39, 40, 42, 43, 44, 53, 54, 55, 57, 59, 60, 61,
      62, 67, 71, 76, 77, 92, 98, 116

V

Vasoactive amines   75
Vidian nerve   107, 118

W

Wedge resection of middle turbinate   65, 73